Counseling for Unplanned Pregnancy and Infertility

RESOURCES FOR
CHRISTIAN COUNSELING

RESOURCES FOR CHRISTIAN COUNSELING

VOLUME TEN

Counseling for Unplanned Pregnancy and Infertility

EVERETT L. WORTHINGTON, Jr., Ph.D.

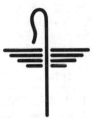

RESOURCES FOR
CHRISTIAN COUNSELING

—————— General Editor ——————

Gary R. Collins, Ph.D.

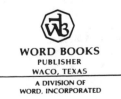

WORD BOOKS
PUBLISHER
WACO, TEXAS
A DIVISION OF
WORD, INCORPORATED

Library of Congress Cataloging-in-Publication Data

Worthington, Everett L., 1946–
　Counseling for unplanned pregnancy and infertility.

　(Resources for Christian counseling ; v. 10)
　Bibliography: p.
　Includes index.
　1. Pregnant women—Pastoral counseling of.　2. Pregnancy, Unwanted—Psychological aspects.　3. Infertility—Patients—Pastoral counseling of.　I. Title.　II. Series.
BV4445.6.W67　1987　　　253.5　　　87-21698
ISBN 0-8499-0588-5

Printed in the United States of America

7898 FG 987654321

To Christen, Jonathan, Becca, and Katy Anna,
our children

"Children are a gift from God; they are his reward."
(Ps. 127:3 LB)

and
to Tom Allport, Jerry Rouse, Buzz Kell, and Doug McMurry,
our pastors

ACKNOWLEDGMENTS

GOD HAS BLESSED KIRBY AND ME WITH FIVE PREGNANCIES—one miscarriage and four living, wonderful children. Each child has been a prayed-for and wanted person. Each is a wonderful blessing. Kirby and I have never had to face the anguish of an unwanted pregnancy. For that we are grateful.

At the time of our first birth, I was in graduate school, looking for a topic for my dissertation research. We had attended Lamaze classes at the University of Missouri-Columbia Hospital and had heard how great the childbirth experience was supposed to be. It conjured up pictures in our minds of sitting casually on the side of the bed playing checkers and sipping lemonade while the baby slipped easily to the bed, rolled over, dressed himself or herself and offered to do some chores around the house. In the end, it wasn't exactly like that. Kirby said it hurt. Imagine that! She even looked like it hurt. At least, she was not like the woman in the other half of the room, shouting, "Get away from me, don't touch me," then ten seconds later screaming, "Where are you? Don't you dare leave me."

Our second birth, two years later, was not much easier. Kirby began to have contractions about six o'clock one evening. We waited a while, then picked up her bag and trundled her off to the hospital.

"A fingertip!" she repeated incredulously to the intern who had just examined her for cervical dilation.

"Look, lady," he said with what he probably considered his best bedside manner, "You are not ready yet. Go home and stay there until the contractions make your eyes cross and take away your breath."

So we picked up her bag and trundled off to home.

Time passed. Kirby was having back labor, which she found was aided greatly if I rubbed the small of her back, just above the base of her spine. I had to rub *hard*, though, putting elbow power into the massage.

About 9:30 she suddenly got a strange look on her face and said, "Unggh"—or something equally as intelligible. Loosely translated that meant, "We'd-better-get-to-the-hospital-if-you-don't-want-to-deliver-this-baby-on-the-living-room-floor." So we (rapidly) picked up her bag and (quickly) trundled toward the hospital.

As we were getting into the car, Kirby said, "Arggh." (I-think-I'm-going-to-push-if-you-don't-rub-my back.) So we stood in the driveway, and I rubbed in big circles with her leaning over on her hands and knees. At every red light, I would rub.

We pulled up in the parking lot of the University Hospital and I leaped out. Kirby rolled out. "Arggh." *Oh, no, not "Arggh" again,* I thought. She dropped to her hands and knees, and I rubbed her lower back.

Naturally, along came three dating couples. "Hmm, kinky," I heard one mutter.

Finally, we arrived at the admissions desk. "Just fill out these forms and have a seat. We'll be with you in a few minutes," said the receptionist.

"Arggh," said Kirby (with some feeling).

"We'll take you right up," said the receptionist after seeing Kirby and me go through our back rubbing routine for about five seconds. Everyone in the waiting room was assiduously examining his or her fingernails.

Up the elevator we went, Kirby in the wheelchair that the hospital insisted on her using. When we arrived at the labor and delivery floor, we headed down the long hall at a good clip.

"Arrrggghhh," (Arggh, and-I-ain't-fooling-around-this-time).

Thump. That was the sound of Kirby bailing out of a moving wheelchair onto her hands and knees. I stood by, rubbing vigorously and looking helplessly at the orderly who was running down the hall yelling, "There's a woman having a baby in the hall." Actually, Jonathan came much later (about ten minutes or so). After that night, we were legendary on campus.

All of this is a roundabout way of thanking Kirby and my children for getting me interested in the area of childbirth. I have since conducted research on pain control in childbirth and on the transition to parenthood, and I have recently begun to study adolescent pregnancy and decisions about adoption versus child rearing for adolescent mothers. The many participants in my research since 1977 have contributed to this book through talking to me about their experiences and through completing endless questionnaires about their experiences.

I also want to thank the undergraduate and graduate students and nurses who have helped with the research over the years. I am particularly indebted to Glen Martin, Michael Shumate, Bev Buston, David Morrow, Melinda Queen, Dale Berry, Cheryl Colecchi, Cynthia Clark, Kathy Barnes, Bela Singha, Ruth Grayberg, Anne Campbell, JoAnne Henry, Judy Collins, and numerous childbirth educators in Richmond. My mother, too, has spent time talking to me about her work as a nurse on an obstetrical ward. Some of the anecdotes in the book are from her experience.

Don Danser, my friend and colleague, directed the Richmond Metropolitan Crisis Pregnancy Center and allowed me to serve as his clinical supervisor and as an advisory board member at the Center. Don has had an enormous impact on my life.

The secretaries in the department of psychology at Virginia Commonwealth University have been patient and forgiving of my many demands. They are prompt, cheerful, efficient, and very professional. Derrick Washington has typed and helped me immeasurably throughout the preparation of this manuscript, and in the many other tasks that I have asked of him. The faculty and administration of the department of psychology have supported me in pursuing this work even if some faculty held differing opinions. I appreciate their openness and fairness.

As with previous books of mine, Rena Canipe has allowed our family to stay at her house and has given of herself while I have been writing. She has also encouraged me to persevere. I am grateful for having known her. She is a wonderful Christian example.

Finally, I want to thank my helpmate. Not just for reading and critiquing the manuscript. Not just for bearing our children. Not just for being my partner in raising our children. Not just for being a wonderful Christian wife, mother, and person—to which anyone who knows her can attest. I want to thank her for all of those, but also for faithfully loving and supporting me, always.

CONTENTS

EDITOR'S PREFACE

I FIRST MET EVERETT WORTHINGTON in a coffeehouse in Washington, D.C., after he had presented an impressive scientific paper before a group of professional colleagues. Quiet and unassuming, Ev quickly impressed me with his warmth, his genuine Christian convictions, his sincere humility and his relaxed sense of humor. I already knew about his encyclopedic knowledge concerning marriage, family, and pregnancy issues—his books and numerous articles demonstrate that repeatedly. What I didn't know until our coffeeshop meeting was that Everett Worthington is also a family man. He knows the joys and challenges of being a parent; and he knows the pain of losing a child. Through his years of counseling experience he has gained an understanding of the pain of infertility and unwanted pregnancies, and the problems of unhealthy children. I can think of no one who is better qualified to write a book on this topic of pregnancy-related issues.

This volume is the tenth in the Resources for Christian Counseling series. All of the authors in this series have been asked to produce clear, practical, up-to-date overviews of the issues faced by contemporary Christian counselors. Written by counseling experts, each of whom has a strong Christian commitment, these books are intended to be examples of accurate psychology and careful use of Scripture. Each has a clear evangelical perspective, careful documentation, a strong practical orientation, and freedom from the sweeping statements and undocumented rhetoric that sometimes characterize books in the counseling field. All of the Resources for Christian Counseling books have similar bindings and together they will comprise a complete encyclopedia of Christian counseling.

The field of Christian counseling is complex, confusing to many people, threatening to some, and increasingly attacked—sometimes with vehemence—by critics within the church and without. In the midst of this controversy individuals and families still struggle with personal problems. Teenagers still get pregnant, stress is still prevalent, and is both a personal and social issue. Many still struggle with the pain of unwanted children, guilt over abortion, the trauma of mentally and physically deformed infants, the grief of miscarriage, the uncertainty of difficult decisions, the agony of failing marriages, and a host of other problems. These don't go away in response to the statements of well-intentioned but ill-informed advice givers. Many people need the guidance that comes from caring, biblically astute, well-informed pastors and other counselors. These books in this series are being prepared with the hope that they will be useful, practical, state-of-the-art Christian counseling guides.

Dr. Worthington has tackled some important, relevant, and painful issues in these pages. Drawing on his biblical knowledge, his counseling expertise, his personal experiences, and his impressive familiarity with the psychological literature, he has written a book that you surely will find useful, sometimes humorous and even fun to read; I am sure it will help you to help others, who face the problems of unplanned pregnancies and infertility.

Gary R. Collins, Ph.D.
Kildeer, Illinois

INTRODUCTION

PEOPLE KEEP HAVING BABIES. Inevitably, some people will not have their babies at the most opportune time. Those women and their families must cope with their unplanned and initially unwanted pregnancies. Unwanted pregnancies can develop into unwanted children, but they need not. Having a baby is more than attending Lamaze classes. It is more than lying on a delivery table while a board of helpers shout, "Push 'im out, push 'im out, waaayy out," in the ear of the mother. It, too, is more than changing a life that was running as smoothly as a gentle stream into a raging, destructive wall of water.

This book is aimed at helpers who are consulted by women and families who are dealing with unplanned pregnancies and with infertility (although research on infertility is only now beginning to be published). As a helper consulted by people in the tyranny of indecision, you need weapons to battle the tyrant. By understanding the causes of the problems, you will gain peace. By understanding how to work with the family, you will gain confidence. By understanding the limits of the usefulness of the helper, you will gain greater faith in Jesus as you see the solutions he can work in the lives of the troubled.

My goals in this book are threefold. First, I want to arm you with understanding and techniques to help those needing to deal with unplanned pregnancies. Second, I want to help you think about ways that the problems might be prevented or lessened with the people in your congregation or with your clientele. Finally, I want to place this great human problem within the context of saving and redeeming faith in Jesus Christ.

This is not a theological study of unplanned pregnancy and infertility, which might begin with God's promise to "increase woman's pain in childbearing," which has filtered down into history as social mores that promote even more anguish than can be captured with a single labor and delivery. It does not propose "spiritual" solutions to problems that are divorced from the social and psychological problems of real humans who must struggle with their pain. It does not just say, "Rely on Jesus," and walk away. Rather, it treats problems as whole problems involving social, psychological, physical, and spiritual elements that cannot be separated, because people cannot separate their emotions, thoughts, or behavior from their faith.

When I began to write this book, I soon realized that I had undertaken a task that seemed too ambitious. I wanted to help *everyone* with problem pregnancies using *all* means of helping that could be used by *every* helper. That task loomed impossible. I had to make some choices of what I wanted to focus my efforts upon if the book were not to be a collection of platitudes.

First, I tried to cover most common types of unplanned pregnancies.

Second, I had to decide whether to focus primarily on individual or family counseling. Despite the many individuals who seek counseling, I elected to emphasize counseling families with unplanned pregnancies. In many instances, counseling will be marriage counseling, for the marriage is where most of the action is. However, in some situations, other family members become important, such as with adolescent pregnancy. When midlife parents who have adolescent children become pregnant, the adolescent is often affected and must be included in the counseling. This is also true if younger children begin to "act out" after it becomes known that the parents are going to have another child.

Third, I had to decide who might benefit from reading the book. There are many types of counselors for whom a book on counseling families with problem pregnancies could be useful. Physicians and nurses who generally break the news to the mother that she is indeed pregnant encounter responses that range all the way from joy to stoic acceptance to full-blown psychotic breaks. Childbirth educators also have the opportunity to counsel with many couples who attend Lamaze or Bradley classes because they think they *should* attend. Through the sensitivity and wisdom of the childbirth educator, many are helped. Counselors in public agencies often deal with those who have unplanned pregnancies. These agencies might include community mental health agencies, crisis pregnancy centers, Planned Parenthood agencies, Catholic Family Services agencies, university counseling centers, and private counseling offices. The philosophies of agency counselors may differ widely—across agencies and even within the same agency. Usually, these counselors care about the pregnant woman and want the best for her. They have the potential to powerfully influence the woman, her family, and their decisions. Private counselors, such as psychiatrists, psychologists, licensed social workers, and licensed counselors also see people with unplanned pregnancies, usually when a serious problem such as depression or threatened divorce complicates the pregnancy. Finally, pastors and pastoral counselors probably do most counseling of families with unplanned pregnancies. In a major review of research on religious counseling,[1] I found that a large majority of the problems that pastors encounter in counseling involve marriage or family concerns.

Fourth, I had to decide how to organize a variety of topics, including areas with a wealth of supportive research and writing (such as adolescent pregnancy), and those with little empirical, supportive research (such as infertility).

This book is targeted at helping in settings that are explicitly Christian. This does not necessarily mean that the clients will be Christian or that all of the counselors will agree on the theory of counseling, their interpretation of Scripture, or even the time of day. Christians, who have a strong concern for absolute truth, often have an overdeveloped sensitivity to perceived error. They frequently disagree. I hope that readers can go beyond the points on which we disagree and still be enriched by the book. I have assumed throughout the book that the reader is an experienced counselor, so I have not written a technique-oriented book. I have tried to provide information about the various types of unplanned pregnancies and point out some ways the counselor might use the information.

The first part of the book deals with how to conceptualize the problem of unplanned pregnancy and with descriptions of ways to help families with unplanned pregnancies. After a brief overview (chapter 1), I focus on the pregnancy as a crisis and a life transition (chapter 2) and describe some ways I do counseling (chapter 3). Although the method I advocate works for me, other counselors might be more effective with other methods of counseling. On the basis of my understanding of life transitions, I predict the likelihood of success of alternative methods of marriage and family counseling for couples in life transitions.

The second part of the book deals with pregnancies that are too early. For example, teenage pregnancies (chapter 4) are discussed—especially the impact of the teen pregnancy on the family of the teen. A second too-early pregnancy is one that occurs before a couple is married, regardless of how old the couple are (chapter 5). Despite the biblical injunction forbidding sexual intercourse before marriage, many couples who are Christians commit this sin and some inevitably become pregnant. If they are not to compound their sin by electing to abort their child, they must deal with the illegitimate pregnancy—either within the context of the church or outside of it. A third pregnancy that is too early is one that occurs early in the marriage while the newly wedded couple are still adjusting to their new life together (chapter 6), and a fourth type is a multiple birth or one occurring soon after another birth (chapter 7). Although the baby may be desired, the timing is seen as difficult because it adds the stress of a new pregnancy to the already considerable stress of adjusting to an infant.

The third part of the book deals with pregnancies that are too late or that never occur. Perhaps the most common might be called "one too many" (chapter 8). We know that, "Lo, sons are a heritage from the Lord . . . like arrows in the hand of a warrior are the sons of one's youth. Happy is a man who has a quiver full of them!" (Ps. 127:3a, 4, 5). What we are not told is what to do when one's quiver runneth over. Sometimes the couple find they have a size 4 quiver when they already have 5 arrows. That requires adjustment. A "one-too-many" pregnancy covered in chapter 8 involves a child who requires special attention from the family—one who is "difficult," mentally retarded, handicapped, or chronically ill. Another too-late pregnancy occurs unexpectedly at the end of the childbearing years (chapter 9). Because many midlife pregnancies end in miscarriage or stillbirth, those difficulties are also covered in that chapter. In chapter 10, I cover the ultimate too-late pregnancy—one that never occurs.

In Part IV of the book, I reflect on ways that writing the book has affected me. There I discuss some of my beliefs about why people suffer, and I affirm the sovereignty of God as the Lord of the universe.

I hope you will evaluate this book as Christian without being preachy and that you will find it practical and theologically true where it addresses theological issues. I hope it will be useful in helping draw both those you help and you closer to the living God.

PART ONE

STRESS, TRANSITIONS, AND FAMILY COUNSELING

CHAPTER ONE

AN OVERVIEW OF UNPLANNED PREGNANCIES

THE SIX CHILDREN GATHERED TOGETHER in the Sunday school room and whispered. At the other end of the table sat an eleven-year-old boy we will call Mikey. He played with his fingers, apparently unaware that the other children were involved in conversation about him. Heads turned toward Mikey and giggles punctuated breathless whispers. Mikey looked up; the other children looked away.

Mikey gazed back at his fingers. A small stream of saliva dripped from his mouth onto the table. More giggles were heard.

In walked Mrs. Johnson, the Sunday school teacher. "Good morning," she said, greeting several children by name. "Happy

Easter." The children stirred and smiled at their beloved teacher. Even Mikey smiled.

It's not easy being retarded, thought Mrs. Johnson. She had often seen the pain of rejection in Mikey's eyes. She couldn't help but notice. His parents seemed to love him, but still they treated him as if he were a ball and chain around their necks. His moderate mental retardation was apparent to the other children, who, while not openly rejecting him, certainly did not include him in their interactions.

"Today, we have a special Easter lesson," explained Mrs. Johnson. "In just a few minutes, I will give you each a large, empty, plastic Easter egg. Then, we'll go outside and spend thirty minutes looking for something to put in the egg that reminds you of Easter. After that, we will come back inside and talk about what we found."

With their eggs in hand, the children rushed excitedly for the door in pairs. Except for Mikey, who went alone.

Thirty minutes later seven secret-bearers regrouped in the classroom. Their eggs, filled with the hidden treasures, were collected within a basket in the center of the table.

Mrs. Johnson extracted the first, and slowly pulled apart the two halves of the plastic shell. Inside was a tiny tree sprout sticking out of a small clump of dirt, and flanked by a split acorn.

"That's mine," boasted Sue, too excited to endure additional suspense.

"How does that remind you of Easter?" asked the teacher.

"That's easy," said Sue. "Easter is a time when we get new life because of Jesus."

Mrs. Johnson selected another egg. As she opened it, a butterfly burst forth and flitted about the room amid squeals and excited laughter. "Whose is this?"

"Mine," said Tab. "Easter is a time when change happens. Like when the butterfly breaks out of his cuckoo."

"You mean 'cocoon,' you dodo bird," said Rachel good-naturedly.

Mrs. Johnson picked up a third egg. She pulled apart the halves, but nothing fell out. It was empty. There was a stunned silence, then the children began whispering to each other.

Shortly all eyes were on Mikey. The children felt betrayed, as if the boy had violated some important social rule. "Mikey did it." "Mikey didn't put nothin' in his." "Come on, Mikey, that's not fair." Like a chorus they accused him.

As Mikey raised his eyes, his face flushed; his accumulated frustration and anger were near the surface. Struggling to find the words to say, at last he shouted, "I'm right. I *am* right."

There was silence. Anger was not characteristic of Mikey.

"I'm right. The tomb *was* empty."

There was a thoughtful silence in the room while Mikey continued: "Jesus went home to God." He began to cry.

Slowly, one of the children rose and walked to the end of the table and put his arm around Mikey. Then another. And another. Mikey was finally a wanted child.

About six months later, Mikey died. During the funeral service, while the pastor gave the eulogy, the rear door of the sanctuary opened. Together, six children walked solemnly down the long aisle. And on the altar they laid an empty Easter egg. Mikey had gone home.

THE CHILDREN

This story is true, to the best of my knowledge, and happened within a church in Washington, D.C.[1] In being passed from person to person, it has probably become distorted. But the pain of the millions of unwanted children—at least unwanted initially—is all too real. Not all unwanted children are as blessed as was Mikey. Some never are wanted.

In families where the adults are more concerned with themselves and their own lives than with the child, an unwanted child might be physically or even sexually abused.[2] The short-term impact of abuse on children is enormous. It involves lowered self-esteem, anxiety, fear, depression, anger, hostility, aggression, and, often, sexually inappropriate behavior. In the long term, the effects are also marked, including depression and self-destructive behavior, a tendency to become an abuser, a tendency toward other types of victimization, anxiety, feelings of isolation, substance abuse, and sexual maladjustment.

In other families concerned with their own pain and their own future, an unwanted child might be aborted. In the

27

United States recently there were 359 abortions for every 1000 live births. For teens, there were 730 abortions for every 1000 live births, and the abortion rate is much higher if the teen is 15 or younger and unmarried.[3]

In still other families, an unwanted child is seen as a jailer who restricts the couple's freedom. It hampers the dating of the adolescent mother. Later, it might tie down the adolescent mother's parents during their retirement years.

An unwanted child can be an economic burden. A young career woman decides to put aside her work for the childhood years, but her resentment grows with each passing year. The welfare mother has little time for the new baby. She receives the government check, but has little energy to devote to child-rearing because she is holding down a low-paying job and trying to raise four children without a father.

An unwanted child can be the source of stress. Back-to-back children pile demands so high that a family is submerged. The family struggles for air, for life itself, trying not to neglect the child.

What of the child? He or she grows up in an atmosphere of rejection. Parents say "we love you," but their nonverbal behavior shouts "we don't want you." This pricks the infant's heart and wounds the preschooler's spirit until the adolescent strikes back, creating pain in a cycle of hurt and rejection that seems to escalate continually.

Not every unwanted child began as an unwanted baby; not every unwanted baby grows into an unwanted child; not every unwanted pregnancy grows into an unwanted baby. Some parents, despite the struggles of adjustment, come to accept and love their child even though the child was conceived at an inopportune or inconvenient time. In that there is hope. Those are some of the people who will come to you for counseling.

WHO WILL SEEK YOUR HELP WITH UNPLANNED PREGNANCIES?

Despite the facts, figures, and theories that populate this book, the book is about *people* and how you can help them. Let me introduce you to some of the people you will meet.

In chapter 4, you will meet Rhonda and Sharon. Rhonda was

a cheerleader and president of her junior class at high school when she became pregnant. She and Tim decided to marry, but after four years, they separated and later divorced. Sharon was fourteen, pregnant and afraid. Her parents took her to a crisis counselor to talk her into an abortion that she didn't want.

Charles and Cathy were Christians, but were living together when Cathy became pregnant. They sought advice from their pastor. People in the congregation were divided in their reactions. Many were judgmental, some were supportive. Charles and Cathy decided to have the child and place it for adoption, but giving up their child proved more difficult than they had anticipated. In chapter 5, you will find how Charles and Cathy fared.

In chapter 6, you will meet people attending classes in preparation for childbirth. They carry pillows everywhere and grown men discuss "choo-choo breathing" without batting an eye. You will also learn how a child can transform your life— changing first the wardrobe and then the eating habits. In chapter 7, on close-together pregnancies, I interview Mrs. Howe who has two infants separated by less than one year. She shows me dramatically how many pressures impinge on her. Chapter 8 is about raising children with special problems. The Evert family, with two teenage girls and a mentally retarded infant, meet the Donaldson family, which has three healthy children and one girl with cerebral palsy. Through their conversations, you'll see how the Everts grow.

Clint and Ann were expecting a child at forty-eight. They experienced battles with their obstetrician and others who recommended abortion. Standing firm, they had the child, but he died shortly after birth. In chapter 9, Father Jim counsels Ann about the loss.

PROBLEMS YOU WILL ENCOUNTER

Thus, a variety of women and their families will seek your help for counseling with unplanned pregnancies. The people you counsel can be individuals, couples, or families throughout the entire family life cycle. Often, the special moral issues that can arise in the counseling of a pregnant teen or of a cohabiting couple can involve members within the church community who take strong positions about how and whether you *should* be counseling certain people. So, the counseling extends into the greater community with other couples and families who are in turmoil, and are angry and judgmental.

Your Clients

The counselor must decide who his or her clientele are. Are they Christians exclusively? Some counselors in private practice have referral networks that provide them with clients from the Christians in the community. The demand for a solid, Christian counselor is great enough that the counselor might never (or rarely) see a client who is not Christian. Other counselors may work for a community agency and may have to deal with whoever walks in the door. There may even be restrictions about sharing one's religious beliefs with the counselees, such as only being able to discuss Christianity if he or she brings it up. Some pastors might feel that they have to restrict their counseling to the members of their congregations and their families, whereas others might feel that they have a duty to counsel the unchurched as well. Some pastors look at counseling as a method of evangelism, while others view it as a ministry to the needy regardless of the person's spiritual condition. These decisions depend on the call of God to individual counselors or pastors.

Decision Making

Counseling involves helping people make decisions. Pregnancy is a marker in people's lives. It is one of the most visible signs of transition from one stage of life to another. During that stage, numerous decisions are made. Some people decide between abortion and keeping the child. Others decide between raising the child and giving it up for adoption. Most decide how to conduct their lives after the birth of the child. The community must decide how it will react to the people.

The counselor facilitates decision making. Sometimes decisions are made in an atmosphere of crisis. At other times decisions are rationally and carefully thought out. Regardless of how they are arrived at, the counselor must be flexible enough to work with his or her clients, despite differences between how the clients make decisions and how the counselor makes decisions, despite differences in what the counselor thinks he or she would do in the place of the client, and what the client actually decides.

Much of your counseling will involve helping people through crises. These crises may be quick and volatile, occurring over a two- or three-day period. Or they may be extended over weeks or months.

Counseling might also help people during the post-decision period for they will inevitably have doubts about the course of their decision. You will have to help them maintain their decisions, or in some cases, evaluate the rightness of their decision and perhaps reverse it (if possible). Post-decision repentance and forgiveness may also be necessary, such as when a girl comes to you after having had an abortion and is now convinced that she has sinned. Helping people through the period after a decision is part of helping people through their difficulties.

Counseling might continue throughout the entire pregnancy. A family of a pregnant teen, who will soon be both an adolescent and a mother, will need the nine months of pregnancy just to work out an approach to their lives from the time of birth onward. The newlywed couple will need help with the adjustments of both marriage and pregnancy.

Counseling might continue past the birth of the child. An older family might have to readjust to the presence of a new infant in their house. The newlywed couple may need substantial counsel to adjust to their relationship together and the baby simultaneously.

Ambivalence and Ambiguity

Counseling families with unplanned pregnancies will also involve dealing with ambivalence and ambiguity. Feelings are not usually "pure." The joy of conception and the pride of creation will be balanced by the insecurity of impending parenthood, and feelings of inadequacy, guilt, and pain. Positive and negative emotions become woven together into a fabric that is complex and difficult to disentangle. Generally, in emotionally loaded situations, many feelings will be fused together.

In politics and in theological discussions, we often simplify issues into essentials. In dealing with people in trouble, however, truth and compassion must be intertwined. Jesus ate with the tax collectors, the prostitutes, and the Pharisees. He did not condone what they did and even at times spoke harshly to them about their calumny. Yet he maintained an open relationship with them which involved acceptance of them as people. Otherwise, why did they continue to associate with him? No one will maintain a voluntary relationship in an atmosphere of judgment and lack of acceptance. That places special demands on counselors, to speak the truth in love, to support the person but be clear about his or her own values. Counselors will need to accept the inherent ambiguities of feelings, but try to point an unambiguous way to Jesus through actions of love and truth.

PREVENTION OF SOME UNPLANNED PREGNANCIES

People are fallen. As part of the consequences of Adam and Eve's choice to willfully sin against God, the pain of childbearing is increased. That pain involves more than the physical discomfort we call labor; it involves the psychological and social costs of childbearing, too. We can never entirely prevent that pain. Yet, as Christians we continually struggle against the effects of the fall. So, we must do our best to ameliorate unnecessary pain in childbearing. There are four areas for our preventive efforts.

Education

We must impart information and values in order to reduce the pain in unplanned pregnancies. I list this first reluctantly. Since the Enlightenment in the eighteenth century, society has looked to education to solve the problems of existence. But education will never solve those problems. It will be especially ineffective within a value-neutral society. For example, sex education within the schools was once seen as the solution to teen pregnancy. After sex education became widespread, the problem not only did not recede, it exploded. One reason for the explosion was that we live in a pluralistic society in which people embrace a multitude of views. In an effort to keep from offending elements of society, value-laden issues of sexuality were presented in a value-neutral manner. Children learned that sexuality could be thought about and practiced apart from morals—or at best, morals were treated as a matter of individual choice. God made sex to be pleasurable. When sex is talked about and practiced in a value-neutral environment, the result should have been entirely predictable. Children, as they grow through adolescence and into young adulthood, will enjoy sex and will engage in it with increasing frequency.

Thus, in the church and in the home we cannot educate people apart from eternal, Judeo-Christian values. Education can be formal or informal, in large groups or small, in sermons or private conversations, in church or in the home.[4] No matter where or how we educate, we must do so in the context of our values.

We can educate people about how to behave if they are pregnant. We can educate people about how to avoid pregnancies through birth control or through chastity. We can educate people about how to deal with temptations to sin and how to delay gratification. We can even educate people about how to cope with problems and difficult decisions when they arise. People can be given information that they have not previously heard and they can be given ways to combat information that argues against Christian values. However, education alone is not enough.

Skill Development

Knowing how one should think about sexual behavior and unplanned pregnancies is not necessarily the same as dealing with them. We must think beyond mere information transmission toward skill development. Sunday school courses that study the biblical position of the family or of morality must be followed by other courses that teach behavioral principles and help people apply the scriptural lessons in their lives. For example, adolescent girls might use role playing to practice ways of saying no to the advances of adolescent boys. Adolescent boys might be told about ways to handle the peer pressure that encourages premarital sex. Then they might practice ways to say no in tempting situations.

33

Newlywed couples might be told about the likely conflicts of the first year of marriage and encouraged to seek a biblical understanding of their roles and behavior within the marriage. That might be followed by role playing about how to argue in love, finding resolutions to difficulties without hurting each other.

Older families might be told about the crises of midlife and the stresses and strains on individuals and on family relationships as the children age. Then, they might be engaged in a family enrichment retreat to work out some of the issues among the family members. Or, financial planning might be needed to handle likely future financial strains, such as financing college for the child or providing retirement income.

Social Support

During times of difficulties, Christians strive to support each other. Friends can be supportive through telephone counseling or face-to-face contact. They can support each other within ongoing Bible study or prayer groups as well as through groups formed for a specific purpose, such as a young mothers group or a new parents group.

But beyond the remedial use of groups to provide social support for the needy,[5] groups can be a source of strength for right behavior that prevents unplanned pregnancies that occur because of sin. Individuals, too, can support right behavior, as can families prominent within the church. The mere presence of happy families encourages those who are struggling.

Political Action

As Moses led the people of Israel away from Egypt, suppose he thought, *Here are a million people under my charge. These people are a diverse group with many different beliefs and values. I can't possibly presume that they should obey the same moral principles. Even if I do, it would not be right to place those principles and laws on each person. Rather, I'll let each person decide what is right.* That would have been a chaotic Israel.

No nation ever thinks that way. All nations impose their views of right and wrong on all the people, whether the people agree or not. In the United States, we do this through elected, representative government. Christians need to be personally involved in all aspects of politics. Prevention of some unplanned pregnancies can be aided through just and sound legislation. For long periods of time, Christians have bought the myth that government should be religiously neutral. It cannot be neutral. Christians should work within the system to promote solid Christian values through law. This does not mean that all Christians will necessarily agree on the issues. Because real-life dilemmas are complex, we tend to emphasize one side of the truth more than another, while another Christian might emphasize the second truth more than the first. Even though on many issues there might not be a universally accepted "Christian" position, Christians must become more involved in politics if we are to prevent many of the tragedies that occur.

Like any of the methods of prevention, political action cannot entirely eliminate the problem. It can only address part of the problem. Nonetheless, political action is a part of the arsenal we have to battle the effects of the fall.[6] Let us use that weapon wisely and sensitively.

CHAPTER TWO

CRISIS AND LIFE TRANSITION

"I SHOULD HAVE SUSPECTED that I was pregnant when I woke up, smiled at Mark who was sleeping blissfully beside me, and then heaved myself out of bed. And the heaving didn't stop there. I heaved all the way to the bathroom. After two days, I broke down and went to the doctor."

Anna continued, mimicking the doctor in a singsong voice. "'Congratulations,' he said to me. 'You're preg. . . .'"

She raised her hand, palm outward, and assumed a stern look. "'Hold it. Remember, before you say anything, the bearer of bad news often loses his own head.'" Anna paused and looked directly at me. "You know what that doctor did?" she asked me. "He yelled for the nurse."

I listened to Anna describe her discovery of the pregnancy. She and Mark were both 49, with a previously well-adjusted fourteen-year-old son, Marco, and a preadolescent ten-year-old daughter, Maria. Hearing her good-natured account of "the annunciation," as she called it, it was hard for me to believe how deeply the whole family had been affected by the recent birth of their new daughter, Ali.

Anna had gone back to work when Maria had entered elementary school so that the family could save money for the college education of the children. Although she said she did not feel fulfilled with her work and (if the truth were known) did not even enjoy it, she did like the extras that the money allowed the family to enjoy. They had bought a trailer on some lake-front property and now owned a speed boat.

Her husband rubbed his hand back over his brown and gray hair and said to me, "You know, Ev, I don't think we've ever recovered from Anna's initial upheaval. We've been listing by 45 degrees from the vertical ever since. We thought that when Ali was born things would get better. It just corrected our list by 90 degrees. Anna, of course, had to quit her work when Ali was born. There was no way that we were going to allow someone else to raise our child.

"Then the bills started to come in. We thought we had misnamed Ali—we should have named her *Bill*. We had thought our family was finished, so I didn't have maternity insurance. The doctors were sympathetic, but sent the bills anyway. Our house payments were dependent on two incomes. Heaven knows, adolescents seem to have to buy every pair of blue jeans that has any new wrinkle or bulge that is different from last week's pair or they will not, God forbid, be 'in.'"

"It sounds as if the pressure was mounting on the whole family," I summarized.

"It sure was," said Anna with a sidelong glance at Marco. "That's when Marco started to have trouble at school. Not too long after Ali was born. He's always been such a good-natured kid, but now it's nothing but fights."

Everyone looked at Marco, who stared sullenly at the floor with his arms folded across his chest. He made no effort to rise to the provocation to defend himself.

37

I cleared my throat. "So I gather that he has been in trouble with the school?"

"Yeah, I've been in trouble with the school. And with the guys. And with the family. Everybody's on my case. I'm just the bad guy."

"So you're the bad guy, huh? Sounds like you think everyone is down on you," I said.

He wiped his hair back in an unconscious imitation of his father. "Yeah. That's what I think. What do you think? You see how they talk about me and look at me. Everyone blames me. I didn't get her pregnant." Marco nodded toward his mother.

"Just watch your mouth, Marco," interrupted Mark angrily.

"Well, I didn't. Now you're off working that extra job and are always away and we don't ever go to the lake anymore. And all of you blame me for everything. I can't go out at nights anymore. I can't have decent clothes. I can't. . . ."

"That's enough, Marco," said Anna. She turned to me. "Well, that's the way it usually is around the house. We're a real nuclear family at least—complete with nuclear explosions."

CRISIS IN THE FAMILY

When we think of a crisis, we usually think of a time of extreme upheaval which soon recedes. As Mark and Anna's family has experienced, though, crises generally take time to stabilize. Numerous changes require adjustment. As often as not, the adjustment also requires adjustment, as Mark described when he said that the birth of the child corrected a 45-degree lean by 90 degrees!

For many, pregnancy is a crisis.[1] Yet each year, millions of people became pregnant without experiencing great turmoil. Why? What predicts whether or not a family will experience a crisis with the pregnancy and birth of a child?

An excellent model for describing family crises has been developed by Reuben Hill (The ABCX Model)[2] and refined by Hamilton McCubbin and Joan Patterson when they were at the University of Minnesota (the Double ABCX Model).[3] These family scholars have been more interested in describing family operation from a systems perspective than in investigating family therapy. Nonetheless, the counselor can learn much by understanding their model.

The ABCX Model identifies three factors that combine to determine whether or not a crisis (X factor) is experienced by a family. These are stressor and hardships (A factor), resources (B factor), and perception of the stressor (C factor).

The stressor (A factor) is any life event that has an impact on the family capable of affecting the family system. For Mark and Anna, both the pregnancy and the birth were stressors. Also part of the A factor are the hardships associated with the stressor. For example, with the birth of the new baby, the financial strains due to purchases of new clothes and paying doctors and hospital bills were associated hardships.

The resources of the family (B factor) include family and other physical and psychological resources. For example, Mark and Anna's accumulated savings and the presence of a social support system such as their close church fellowship were resources on which they drew.

The family's perception of the stressor (C factor) is important to determining the family's reaction to the stressor. If the family views the stressor and the associated hardships as overwhelming, they will be overwhelmed. If the family views the stressor as a challenge, they will be challenged. The view of the stressor will not change the severity of the stressor, but it will affect the family's response to it. One of Mark and Anna's strong family resources is their humor. Despite their hardships, they can see the humor and irony in life, which not only keeps their mood high, but opens them up for unexpected solutions.

Crisis (X factor) is the amount of disruption experienced by a family, based on the interaction of the stressor and hardships, the family resources, and the perception of the stressor. Crisis is best thought of as being present to some degree in all life transitions. The degree of crisis affects the ways the family copes with it.

Most crises do not appear instantaneously and disappear suddenly; rather, crises occur over some length of time. During that time the family tries to adapt to the crisis. The degree of adaptation is described by McCubbin and Patterson as the Double ABCX Model. Hill's ABCX Model describes the precrisis state, whereas the Double ABCX Model adds a consideration of the family's coping attempts after the crisis has begun. How well the family adapts to the crisis (xX factor) depends on the pileup of other stressors (aA factor), the existing and new resources (bB factor), and the ongoing perception of the crisis (cC factor).

Transitions rarely come singly in neat progression. They often pile up (aA factor). For example, Mark and Anna's new child appeared as Marco was struggling with adolescence. Anna had to quit work and assume a role she thought she was finished with—caretaker of an infant. Mark took a second job and the whole family had to pull back on their spending. To add to the stress even further, their leisure activity was drastically changed. A personal example drove this point home for me. When our fourth child was born, several stressors occurred in rapid succession. Katy Anna could hear only the loudest sounds. The first months were marked by uncertainty over the extent of her hearing difficulty and involved several visits to hearing specialists. At eight months, God miraculously healed her with no hearing loss at all. At the same time, I was being considered for promotion and tenure at work, which resulted in my spending considerable energy evaluating my career and seeking God's direction for the upcoming seven or so years. Kirby had become anemic, making her tired and listless beyond the normal parental tiredness associated with infants. To complicate matters, our church changed pastors; Kirby questioned her ability to cope with four children, three of whom were preschoolers; and one goldfish leaped from its tank in a dramatic suicidal gesture.

During a period of crisis, the family draws upon its resources and tries to establish new resources (bB factor). The personal strengths of family members are tested as well as the solidity of the family and of the marriage. Finally, the social support system is taxed. For instance, in Mark and Anna's family, Mark took on a second job to create additional financial resources to maintain the family's style of life. As the family tried to retrench to less luxurious living, their conflict increased, both within the family and between Marco and his peers.

Throughout the crisis period, the family also struggles to

make sense of their difficulties (cC factor). They continually search for causes of the problems they are having and they seek meaning in their troubles. This is a time when many people turn to Jesus for help. In fact, Olson, McCubbin et al., in a study of a large national sample of Lutheran church members, showed that the most helpful aid to family adaptation was a reliance on their faith.[4]

Adaptation (xX factor) is the way that the family system reorganizes to use its resources and meet the demands of the crisis. This often involves restructuring the family roles, boundaries, and interactions. Adaptation may move the family toward a more flexible and stronger system or toward a more rigid and brittle system. Mark and Anna found later that many changes were necessary in the way their family had been organized. For example, Mark had to increase his involvement in the family while Anna had to stop using humor as much to smooth over conflicts. Both Mark and Anna found it necessary to give more freedom to Marco, who also became more involved with family life. Marco was allowed to take some part-time jobs to earn his own extra spending money.

The Double ABCX Model of crisis is a sophisticated analysis of the stresses and strains on the family during stressful periods. In this brief synopsis, I can only hope to have discussed the high spots. For the marriage and family counselor, understanding this model can greatly aid in conceptualization of the family under stress.

Understanding this model helps counselors gain appreciation for the complexity of a crisis and for the variety of naturally occurring aids to the family for getting past the crisis. The counselor is an important resource for the family, but only one resource among many. The counselor must alertly involve the family with other resources and other members of the loving community to help them successfully adapt to their crisis.

LIFE TRANSITIONS IN THE FAMILY

Since Freud discussed the oral, anal, phallic, latency, and mature genital stages of psychological development, numerous writers have described predictable stages individuals supposedly go through. Erickson described eight stages of psychosocial development based on the theories of Freud. Piaget described stages through which children develop their thinking until they reach the capacity to reason maturely. Perry described stages through which college students and other adults develop their intellectual and ethical reasoning. Kohlberg has described six stages of moral development through which children and adults supposedly progress.[5]

Stages in the Family Life Cycle

Other writers have applied the notion of predictable stages to life in the family. Perhaps the best known of the family life-cycle theorists is Duvall[6] who divided the family into four parts and eight stages. She marked the onset of each new stage with a significant life transition.

Early in the development of thinking about the family life cycle, the emphasis was on describing a family's tasks and events within each stage. Recently, a different type of theory has gained ascendancy. Instead of describing what happens *during* a stage, theorists have turned their attention to what happens as the family moves from one stage to another; in other words, life transitions. Attention was drawn to life transitions by the publishing of Gail Sheehy's best seller, *Passages*, which describes the crises that occur around common life transitions.[7]

The Importance of Life Transitions

Clearly, how families live during the stable times of their lives is of great importance. One assumption that seems reasonable, though, is that when a family is operating stably, only some life event that is disruptive will move the family to a different way of living. That life event can be a normative one—that is, an event most people experience—such as when a couple has their first child. Or, the life event can be non-normative—one experienced by relatively few people—such as when a teenager becomes pregnant before marriage.

The question that has intrigued me for years is, why some families experience normative or non-normative transitions and handle them smoothly while other families experience similar transitions and fall apart.

CHARACTERISTICS OF LIFE EVENTS

The Double ABCX Model of crisis explains some of the factors that might answer that question, but the answers are not very specific. Some of the scholars who have studied life transitions shed some light on the question. For example, Danish, Smyer, and Nowak summarized six characteristics of life events that affect how individuals react to them.[8]

1. *Timing.* Whether the event occurs on time, earlier than expected, or later than expected influences the person's reaction to the event. This is easy to see with unplanned pregnancies. I have even organized this book in terms of when, relative to expectations, pregnancies occur—too early or too late.

2. *Duration.* The duration of a transition also affects the response of the person to the transition. For example, pregnancy helps a couple anticipate the birth of the child. The nine months help them adjust to the new addition. (Nine months' waiting period also is God's method of birth control, since the blissfully unsuspecting couple might be so enthralled with the pregnancy and the thought of having children that they might create about twenty in short order if they didn't have to wait nine months minimum between each decision to add to their family.[9]) It is easy to see how pregnancies that don't last long enough and those that last too long are stressful. Many mothers think that nine months *is* too long.

3. *Sequencing.* When events occur out of their expected order, the family has difficulty adjusting to the event. When pregnancy precedes marriage, the family does not usually cope as well with the pregnancy as when it occurs in the more expected order.

4. *Cohort specificity.* Each generation has its own norms that govern behavior. A family of ten was not uncommon in 1888 but would be a strain in 1988.

5. *Probability of the occurrence of the event.* Events that are statistically rare are generally more stressful for the family than are events that are more common. For instance, when a family has a child that is deformed or chronically ill, that family finds little support in dealing with the unique stresses of that event.

43

——————————

6. *Contextual purity of the event.* Events that occur in isolation from other stresses are more easily coped with than events that pile up. Thus, the family with three children spaced four years apart will generally react in a less volatile manner than the family with an infant followed nine months later by the birth of twins. Stressful events that occur close together in time often produce reactions that are more extreme than the sum of the reactions they might have produced separately.

CHARACTERISTICS OF THE FAMILY

Besides the characteristics of the events, three other factors especially affect the family's responses to transitions: the amount of disruption in the family's time schedules, the number of new decisions in which family members disagree initially, and the amount of instability in the family power structure prior to the transitions. I was led to these variables through reviewing the large amount of research on the effects on marriage of the transition to parenthood.[10] The following sections explain these three variables, using one life transition—the transition to parenthood—as an example.

Disruption of Family Members' Time Schedules

When a family member becomes pregnant, time schedules often must be drastically rearranged. Many researchers have documented this.[11] Each individual in the family is affected differently. Some individuals might find the new time schedule more to their liking than the previous one; others find the new time schedule less pleasant, if for no other reason than it is different than what they were used to.

There are a number of reasons why the disruption of time schedules can affect the family members. First, new time schedules force the family to change their ways of meeting their needs for intimacy and distance (time alone). Alexander and his colleagues in their functional family therapy[12] assume that each of a person's activities meets some need for intimacy or distance. Some activities meet needs for intimacy—such as discussing one's values, sharing plans and dreams, experiencing emotions together, and making love. Other activities promote distance. Those activities are ones that isolate the person psychologically or physically. Reading, studying, going fishing alone, or working late each promote distance. Some activities serve an intermediate function. They are coactive, regulating closeness somewhere between distance and intimacy, such as when a couple discusses the events of their day or when a family has a picnic.

Presumably, people attempt to arrange their lives to meet their needs for intimacy, distance and coaction. They are usually satisfied if their needs are close to, if not exactly, met. For example, let's return to Mark and Anna's family. Mark and Anna are both sociable people. They are comfortable having lots of coaction and intimacy and try to limit the amount of distancing they do. When Mark had to take a second job, he no longer could interact with his family the way he did prior to the birth of the new child. The times of relaxing socialization at the lake were discarded, and instead Mark worked as a night watchman. He soon became starved for social interaction. At the same time, Marco missed the times of family intimacy and—though he probably did not do it intentionally—he began to have difficulties at school, which forced his parents to interact more with him. Of course, he didn't always like the types of interactions he was having, but any interaction was better than none. Anna, who had perhaps the greatest social needs in the family, experienced the greatest disruption in her time schedule. Instead of enjoying the company of the gregarious professionals she worked with in her real estate office, she found herself trying to relate meaningfully to dirty diapers and spit-up. Besides missing the social interaction at work, she also missed the family intimacy. Each family member experienced a substantial disruption in his or her time schedule, and it took months before they could rearrange their activities so that they were not continually miserable.

A life transition might affect time schedules greatly, some, or not at all. Generally, the more time schedules are disrupted, the more people are distressed by the transition. As they pass through the transition, they try to bring the balance of intimacy, coaction and distance back to where they are comfortable. The ability to accomplish this is determined by a person's resourcefulness in initiating changes, the flexibility of previous time commitments, and the reactions of people inside and out-side of the family to attempts to readjust time schedules.

A second reason that disruption in a person's time schedules produces distress during transitions is because new roles must be assumed. For example, Anna had to resume a role she thought she was finished with—caretaker of an infant. Mark also found that he had to discipline Marco more frequently, because of Marco's reaction to the transition. Maria, the pre-adolescent ten-year-old, gleefully assumed the role of big sis-ter. For her, the elimination of the weekends at the lake were easily compensated for by her being allowed to play with and take care of the baby.

The third reason that changing times schedules affect the family is that *change* is necessary. Most people perceive change to be taxing at best or generally unpleasant. It is not easy to uproot one's established habits and begin afresh. The uncer-tainty of change breeds apprehension. People often prefer the certain misery they know to the misery of uncertainty.

One additional reason that changing time schedules con-tributes to distress during transitions is that parenthood usu-ally increases the number of roles that each family member performs. That is called role strain, which causes people to feel that time is scarce. The addition of extra roles to an already full time schedule makes social time seem scarce because it calls attention to smaller units of time, making family members more aware about how each unit of time is used. For example, a convict in solitary confinement usually does not notice pass-ing minutes, but an executive in multiple roles is aware of the preciousness of each second.

New Decisions Involving Initial Disagreement

A second occurrence during the transition to parenthood is an increase in conflict.[13] Although not all families have more conflict during life transitions, many do.

Each life transition requires new decisions. For example, when a first child is born, the new mother and father must decide such things as (a) who feeds the infant and when, (b) how much to let the infant cry before picking him or her up, (c) what color to paint the infant's room, (d) who will be spit up on before church on Sunday (usually it is the one with the most navy blue on), (e) who changes the dirty diapers, (f) how much the in-laws will be involved in baby-sitting and in child-rearing decisions, (g) how much cuddling the infant will receive, (h) whether to use a pacifier, (i) whether to read Dr. Spock, (j) and how to talk with the youngster (do the parents say, "Ums want-ums blankey?" or "If you were a precocious kid, you would cover yourself with that blanket I have placed to your right."). Some new parents also try to decide how to discipline the child, whether the boy will be allowed to drive at sixteen, and what the curfew will be during college, but most couples delay those decisions until a little later, such as when they are disagreeing over how to discipline their two-year-old.

Because most parents were also raised in families—families that were different from each other—they both observed their parents make decisions during their own childhoods. They usually had strong reactions to the child-rearing methods of their parents. When those reactions differ from the reactions of their spouse, there is often a small nuclear war in the household.

Even more subtle, though, are the observations that were made and were never questioned by the children-now-grown-up. Those decisions are *assumed* to be the only sensible way to behave with the infant. If those assumptions differ from those of the spouse, then a medium-sized nuclear war can erupt within the family.

"Don't pick her up so much, Darling, you'll spoil her rotten," the new mother begins sweetly.

"Ah, now, honey. She's already love-starved. Just look at her. See, she needs to be held." He grins at his bride.

Because both new parents hold different fundamental assumptions about how much to hold the baby, the discussion passes in a neat progression from the honey-sweety stage to the poignant discussion about whether the mother-in-law wears combat boots. In couples who never resolved some of the other fundamental issues of their relationship, the first sentence can lead directly to the mother-in-law problem without even going through the discussion of whether to roll or squeeze the toothpaste tube or whether the toilet seat should be up or down during the night.

Haley described the dynamics of relationships *as if* relationships were governed by rules.[14] He identified three types of rules. Overt rules are those that families explicitly agree upon. Covert rules are patterns of behavior that would be agreed upon if the family were aware of the pattern. Power rules describe who has the power to make decisions within the family and how the decisions were made. When arguments occur, they are usually over who can make the decision. These rules are described as the pragmatics of communication.[15] When family members disagree about who has the power to make decisions, observers usually describe their interactions as a "power struggle." Everyone spends energy rehearsing conversations in their minds and everyone feels as if his or her basic rights are being violated.

When a transition occurs, new decisions are necessary. If there is fundamental agreement about the new decisions because of the backgrounds of the family members, then the family is likely to pass easily through the transition. But if family members are at fundamental loggerheads about the new decisions, then the power rules are tested. Each time a new decision is made, it redefines either greatly or minutely the power rules in the family. If the family initially disagrees about many decisions, then it is likely that the transition will provoke more turmoil than if few decisions require family members to resolve disagreements.

Instability in the Family Power Structure
Prior to the Transitions

Some families have stable power structures. The family with an unstable power structure might be one that is brittle or one that is so shapeless that it appears chaotic.[16] In families with stable power structures, conflicts are usually quickly smoothed out. In families with unstable power structures, conflicts usually grow.

Generally, studies have found that couples who have good relationships prior to parenthood will have good relationships after having their child, but couples who have troubles prior to the child have even worse problems after the birth of the child.[17] Although it is not foolproof, lots of conflict prior to pregnancy usually means the power structure is unstable.

HOW FAMILIES RESPOND TO TRANSITIONS

We might expect families with differences in (a) disruption of their time schedules, (b) number of new decisions that they initially disagree about, and (c) instability of the pre-transition power structure to differ in their response to the transition. They do. Each family characteristic is thought to affect the family differently. Disruptions in time schedules are thought to produce large dislocations in family relationships that require many adjustments over time and give and take among family members as each reacts to the attempts of the others to restructure their roles and time commitments. New decisions involving initial disagreement are thought to produce discrete arguments (or "discussions" as many families like to describe them). These conflicts rise and fall quickly (relative to the time necessary to completely restructure the time schedules of the family). Instability in the family power structure should be expected to produce three effects: an increasing number of discrete conflicts as the power rules become more openly contested, use of increasingly coercive compliance-gaining strategies as family members try harder to get their way, and an increasing dissatisfaction with family life. Families with stable power structures are likely to experience a return to normality quickly (called negative feedback). Families with unstable power structures, though, are likely to have conflicts that increase in proximity, intensity and acrimony.

MARK AND ANNA'S FAMILY REVISITED

In our brief observation of Mark and Anna's family thus far, we might try to understand them by assessing their response to their surprise pregnancy coupled with Marco's transition into full-blown adolescence. The first thing we notice is that their time schedules are greatly changed from prior to the transitions. Mark is working two jobs instead of one. Anna is caring for the infant instead of working in a highly social real estate agency. The whole family is unable to vacation at the lake on weekends. They have tried to make adjustments in their time schedules, but each adjustment has provoked the need for someone else to make adjustments.

Their patterns of conflict demonstrate that Mark and Anna are generally in agreement. We might expect that because they have raised two other children and have made most of the basic decisions about how to care for infants. On the other hand, they are encountering an adolescent for the first time and are thus faced with many new decisions about how to relate to their adolescent son. From the brief interactions we observed, they demonstrate fundamental agreement on the issues, but there are many other issues that are potential difficulties. To determine the extent of their conflict, we would need to observe them discuss other decisions about how to handle Marco. The patterns of conflict between the parents and Marco are more apparent. Marco has begun to challenge his parents openly, indicating that the fundamental power structure within the family is undergoing challenge. This is a normal part of having a child reach adolescence, but causes turmoil nonetheless. Over time, a new power structure will emerge.

From their interactions, it appears that the family has basic stability in power structure. Although change is expected, it will probably evolve as the parents voluntarily relinquish power to Marco to make responsible decisions while Marco demands (probably) more power and autonomy than his parents are eager to give up. Thus, Mark and Anna's family life will probably be characterized by turmoil while they stabilize their time commitments and adjust their needs for intimacy, but it should eventually result in a fairly high functioning family.

CHAPTER THREE

COUNSELING FAMILIES DURING TRANSITIONS

No METHOD OF COUNSELING WORKS ALL THE TIME for all families, not even mine. How we all wish otherwise. We long for some way to take away the pain from every person who asks us for help.

When psychotherapy was first formulated, the founders of various theories made fantastic claims for their methods. They believed that everyone treated by their method would improve. Don Kiesler called this the "uniformity myth."[1] Research has consistently shown that while psychotherapy is clearly more effective than no formal psychotherapy or mere support and attention, it is not effective for all clients. Recently, new research on the effectiveness of psychotherapy has replaced the uniformity myth with the non-uniformity hypothesis[2]: "Which treatments apply to which clinical problems for what persons and under what conditions."[3]

Family counseling, a newer field than individual psychotherapy, has yet to embrace wholeheartedly the non-uniformity hypothesis. Many family therapists still feel (or at least talk) as if their method of counseling will be effective for everyone.

We need to identify several crucial decisions about what kind of family counseling to employ. Then we will briefly examine several well-known theories of family counseling. Most pastors and mental health professionals have a distinct preference for a particular theory of family counseling. Rather than try to convince anyone that my recommendations are better, I will make some predictions about which theories of family counseling are most likely to succeed with families who have (1) disruptions in time schedules, (2) conflict, and (3) instability in their power structure.

Following that, I will identify my beliefs about counseling and discuss guidelines for effective family counseling in the case of unplanned pregnancies. I will conclude by summarizing the stages through which helping relationships pass.

CRUCIAL DECISIONS ABOUT FAMILY COUNSELING

Pastors and other Christian counselors want to give godly counsel. They want to be *Christian* counselors. However, there are important differences among pastors and Christian mental health professionals about (1) what Christian counseling is, (2) how much to use in counseling techniques derived from Christian worship, and (3) how to decide on one's own *style* of counseling.

Christian Counseling

In an earlier book, I defined Christian helping as "helping that is done by a Christian who adheres to Christian assumptions, who relies on Christ as the center of the helping relationship and who uses whatever knowledge God has revealed."[4] Not every Christian would agree with that definition, but for me it makes the important distinction between counselors who happen to be Christians and people who do Christian counseling.

In fact, in a review of empirical research on religious counseling, I identify three views of religious counseling.[5] In one view, Christian counseling is not defined by which technique is used. Since Christian counseling aims at promoting the client's Christian world view, secular counseling techniques might be used exclusively. The goal is to help a person be more fully human and more fully able to appreciate God. Concepts of Christianity might never be discussed in this type of counseling, yet the counselor believes that he or she is doing Christian counseling.

In a second view, Christian counseling uses techniques also commonly used in religious practice. For example, the Christian counselor would recommend such practices as Bible memory, prayer, laying on of hands, confession, songs of praise, scriptural exegesis, or anointing with oil as the basis for counseling.

A third approach to Christian counseling is to use secular counseling techniques that have Christian content. For example, a cognitive therapist might use methods developed by Ellis or Beck or Meichenbaum to explore the beliefs, values, and thoughts of Christian clients. The counselor and client would talk freely about Christian beliefs, values, and behavior but the *techniques* of counseling would come from secular theories of counseling. Techniques of specifically religious practice might or might not be used, depending on the beliefs of the counselor.

Obviously, few approaches to Christian counseling are purely one type. I usually use the third type, while still employing prayer, Scripture, and other explicitly Christian practices when I believe them to be appropriate.

Each counselor must decide how much to use explicitly Christian practices in a counseling session. This depends partly on the beliefs and expectations of the clients and partly on the beliefs of the counselor. Counselors must speak in a language that their clients can understand while remaining true to their own beliefs.

Once a counselor decides how much he or she wants to use spiritual and worship practices directly in counseling, he or she then needs to decide what style of counseling to employ to get biblical counsel across to the counselee. This involves answering a series of questions about how we will work with families.

Who Are Your Clients?

To some extent we are limited in our choice of counselees to whomever comes to us for help. We can shape the general flow of such persons by talking to our usual referral sources, but there are always times when counselees come who are not like our usual ones. By working with those or by referring them to another professional we also shape our future counseling load. Sometimes case loads will simply evolve without our conscious choice. In other instances we may decide that we want to limit our practice—perhaps to members of our congregation, believing Christians, people with marital difficulties, or individuals seeking help generally. We must follow God's leading in shaping our caseload. I believe in thoughtfully and intentionally limiting my caseload, while leaving room for God to intervene sovereignly by bringing someone to me that he has prepared especially for what I can provide.

Still, there is more to shaping our caseload than merely counseling whomever we select or whomever walks through our door. Once we see a person, couple, or family, we can try to change the definition of who has the problem. For example, if a pregnant adolescent were to approach you for counseling, you might want to change the definition of the problem from an individual problem to a family problem. You might or might not be able to convince the girl to invite her parents to counseling, but the definition of who you assume the client(s) to be is up to you. Even if the girl's parents refused to attend counseling with her, you might still think of the family as being the client.

It is possible to engage in this mental hocus-pocus because problems are generally very complex and affect a person's entire social network. You can usually find plenty of evidence to justify family counseling.

We must keep in mind that counseling will usually give our clients a feeling of power, which can be either beneficial or harmful. If you always see individual clients, they will tend to be strengthened—sometimes at the expense of the marriage or family. For example, one woman involved in a difficult marriage attended individual counseling. Whenever she complained about her marriage, her therapist would say, "What do you *want* to do?" She usually would answer that she wanted her husband to be more considerate, to which the therapist might reply, "What do you think is best for *you?*" The implicit message in this therapy is that the individual client is the most important element—what she wants. After months of that onslaught, she "realized" that she did not "want" to be in a painful relationship with her husband. She initiated divorce proceedings.

Imagine what might have happened if that woman had been attending marriage counseling with her husband. The counselor would have been less concerned with what each spouse wanted for himself or herself. Rather, the question that would have guided therapy would more likely have been, how can each of you make a better marriage?

Goals of Counseling

Although there are several levels of goals, in the most fundamental sense, the goal of counseling can be understood as either to solve problems or to promote growth.[6] Problem solving concentrates on relieving the distress and returning people to adaptive living. Counselees might exit counseling better off than they were before the problem, but the main goal is to ameliorate the problem. The alternative goal is to help counselees become better off than they were before counseling. There will be more emphasis on what the counselor thinks is *growth.*

Let's illustrate this with Mark and Anna's family. Suppose they had gone to a counselor who was totally oriented to problem solving. That counselor might focus quickly on the disrupted time schedules of the family members and would single-mindedly pursue changing the time schedules systematically until the family was no longer distressed. He or she might also help Mark and Anna manage their conflicts with Marco in a more productive way. When Christianity is mentioned, it is considered as a way of solving the specific problems that concern Mark and Anna.

Suppose they had gone to a counselor who was totally oriented to growth. That counselor might be concerned about the spiritual relationship of each family member. He or she might try to help each one build a firmer relationship with Christ. The assumption would be that the problems will subside if the proper relationship with Christ exists; therefore, little attention would be given specifically to the unplanned pregnancy and its effects. A different growth-oriented therapist might have assumed that if the family was in turmoil then it must be because their communication was poor. That counselor might try to teach the couple better communication with each other and with Marco. The assumption is the same—if they are able to improve their communication then they will be able to work out any problems that they have with the unplanned pregnancy.

Most counselors are somewhere between these two extremes. They are concerned both with solving problems and with growth of the family. It is usually better for the counselor to decide intentionally how much to emphasize growth or problem-solving than to leave the emphasis unexamined. If no decision is made, counseling often flounders.

Proactive or Reactive

Some counselors plan their counseling and enter each session with an objective. These counselors are proactive. Other counselors like to wait for the counselee to make a move and then react to it. These are reactive. Both styles are potentially effective, provided the counselor remains both flexible and goal directed.

The danger for the proactive counselor is that his or her plan will rule counseling regardless of what the counselees do or say. The proactive counselor must be vigilantly sensitive to the counselee.

The danger for the reactive counselor is that counseling will meander aimlessly. The reactive counselor must keep in mind an ultimate goal and, despite the clients' tangents, continually redirect them toward the goal.

Compliance or Resistance

Counseling is generally aimed at stimulating people either to comply with the suggestions of the counselor who will presumably guide them positively, or to resist the counselor, in which case the counselor can use the resistance to provoke positive change.

Theories of counseling that promote compliance are generally based on cooperation. The counselors give *reasons* for whatever they ask clients to do. They try to help clients learn the principles of behavior change so they can act as their own therapists with future problems. Their approach appeals to the clients' reasonableness.

Resistance-provoking counselors often make unexplained demands, interpret behavior, or give paradoxical directives (asking clients to do the opposite of what is actually desired in a "reverse psychology" approach). Resistance-engendering approaches usually appeal to the clients' emotions.

In-Session or Out-of-Session Behavior

Some approaches to counseling focus on what occurs during the counseling hour. Generally, this is supposed to be a significant hour in the counselee's life and the therapist is supposed to be important to the counselee. Counseling is viewed as very influential.

In other approaches, a counseling session is viewed as merely one of the 168 hours of the week. Change is supposed to occur, if at all, only if counselees apply what they learn from the counseling hour and change their behavior during the rest of the week. Each counseling session focuses on what people do outside of counseling, both what has been done in the past week and what they intend to do in the forthcoming week.

Communication Training

Most family counseling involves some training in communication. But communication training is not as straightforward as it sounds. There are three aspects of communication.

Some counselors focus on the meanings of communication. They will ask questions of family members such as, "What did he just say to you?" or "What do you think she meant by that?" The meanings of nonverbal communication might also be explored. For instance, the counselor might say, "When he clams up after an argument breaks out, what do you think he is thinking?"

Other counselors emphasize interruptions in dialogue. They will say to family members such things as, "Are you aware that you interrupted her before she finished telling you about her concerns?" or "It seems that when a disagreement begins the temperature rises in the exchanges until it becomes threatening; then one of you cools it down with a joke."

Still other counselors are primarily concerned about what communication reveals of the power relationships among family members. They will observe, "When you get angry and raise your voice it seems to inhibit conversation. That's a very powerful way to control the conversation around home." Or, "When you order him to 'be spontaneous,' it really puts him in a bind. If he acts spontaneous, you never can be sure if it's because he is spontaneous or because he is following your orders." These counselors look for the underlying power structure revealed by a communication.

Any communication has all three aspects—meaning, interruptions, and power. The counselor can choose what he or she will pay attention to. Generally it is not possible—and if so, would be tedious and boring—to attend to all three aspects of every communication, so the counselor needs to understand clearly what part of the communication is likely to be most fruitful.

Communication training also involves how frequently the counselor will interrupt the family in order to comment on or correct their communication. Some counselors interrupt frequently, every sentence or two. They want to be sure that family members understand precisely what is being communicated or how to communicate precisely. Other counselors will interrupt less frequently, because the function of communication in terms of power relationships can be most easily seen within longer periods of communication.

Yet counselor preferences in communication training must be balanced with the family's style of communication. Some families are such active communicators that the counselor feels as if he or she is in the room with a runaway locomotive. Those families must generally be interrupted frequently if the counselor is to maintain some semblance of control over the session. For the reticent family, the counselor might want to avoid any interruption until the conversation trickles out on its own accord.

Applying These Decisions to Your Counseling

As with all of the decisions that must be made about how to counsel, I believe they are best made intentionally by the counselor. They should blend together into a style that is compatible with the counselor's personality and with the counselees' problems.

So often counselors counsel as they do because it is fun or because they were trained to counsel in that way, even though their counseling is neither effective nor suited to their counselees. The most effective counseling matches counselees' needs with counselor styles.

MY THEORETICAL PREFERENCES

I think most family problems are due to faulty structures within the family. These faulty structures are unhelpful alliances of power—mother against father, mother and daughter against father, grandparents and child against parents, or even husband and pastor against wife (to name only a few of these unhelpful alliances). Usually alliances are identified by observing communication patterns. So I attempt to change family structures by changing the ways that people communicate and act with each other. I closely identify with the planfulness of Haley's strategic therapy.[7] In conceptualization, Minuchin's structural family therapy is most compatible with my thinking.[8] In method, however, I use more compliance-gaining techniques than Haley or Minuchin and almost never use paradoxical techniques, which direct counselees to do one thing while hoping they do or think the opposite. I appeal to reason and understanding in order to motivate family members to cooperate with my suggestions; this is most closely associated with the behavioral approach to therapy.[9] Thus, if I had to label my particular brand of integration of family therapies, I would describe it as cognitive-behavioral-strategic-structural family therapy. (I almost named it "hyphenated" family therapy.)

If given the choice, I like to meet with the entire family so that the interactions among family members can be easily observed, but in practice I have found that whole families are not always eager to attend family therapy. I thus attend to individuals within the family more than most strict family therapists. I am concerned about their thoughts, emotions, and behaviors both within the family and when they are apart from other family members.

I like to be active during counseling, moving people around and controlling their actions and conversations as much as possible. I have found that families can usually overpower the meek, mild-mannered counselor, so I don my metaphorical super-leader cape when I enter the counseling room. When I work with couples, I am still somewhat directive. With individuals, I am softer in my leadership and appear more empathic and warm.

I believe that clients change because of what they do between counseling sessions, so I use the counseling hour to discuss the "homework" of the previous week and to plan what the family will do between sessions. Each session is used to create dramatic events that will help the family change their behavior before the next one.

Like the "big event" of the Super Bowl or basketball's Final Four or the "Roots" miniseries that captures the attention of the nation throughout the entire two weeks prior to the big event, counseling should be dramatic enough to capture the attention of family members and engage them in trying to change their behavior.

Another way of saying this is to describe a counseling session as the punctuation in the story of life. Sometimes a comma is the only punctuation that is called for, merely a pause to reflect on what is happening. At other times, the counselor needs to set off (an important) part of life by parentheses—or more dramatically by dashes. This defines that portion of the clients' lives as being unusual, set off from the rest of life. Sometimes the counseling session provides a period. Old behaviors must come to a halt. Period. A new thought must begin. At other times the counseling session can be the end of a paragraph or even the beginning of a new section of a story.

Whatever the function, each session of counseling provides some punctuation for the life story of the people you see.

STAGES OF COUNSELING

In earlier work, I have identified five stages that any counseling or helping relationship passes through.[10] In the first stage, a counselor must enter the counselee's world from the counselee's point of view, understanding how he or she subjectively perceives the problem and communicating that the counselor understands the problem.

The second stage, which can actually take place at the same time as the first, involves a counselor in helping a person rethink the problem. People try to make sense of what is happening to them. Based on their understanding of the problem, they try to solve it. Usually, they do not come to pastors or mental health professionals unless their understanding of the problem is not leading to effective solutions. Thus, a counselor must do more than merely help people clarify their thoughts. An effective counselor must help them understand the problem in a *new* way.

Usually, counselors will understand the problem according to their theory. All counselors have a theory whether they realize it or not. Those beliefs about the "real causes" of the problems will guide them in asking questions and in finding information pertinent to solving people's problems. One of the difficulties in helping people rethink their problems is arriving at a clear reconceptualization of the problem. Even more difficult, though, is getting the new understanding out of the counselor's head and into the counselee's mind. To do this requires real counseling skill—skill that is not usually developed until counselors have counseled for two or three years at the minimum.

The third stage of helping is to develop action plans based

61

on the new understanding of the problem. Counselees must be involved in the planning. Depending on counselors' styles, this may be done more or less directly. After action plans are formed, the real work of counseling occurs. The counselees must use the plans outside of the counseling hour.

In the fourth stage of counseling, counselors must support their counselees' attempts to change. If the attempts are successful, counselors help them understand why the attempts succeeded. And if the attempts are unsuccessful, counselors help their people figure out how to change the attempts to make them successful. If the attempts are made only half-heartedly or not at all, counselors help them decide why the rewards of doing the behavior were not strong enough to motivate them to do it. Together, they need to increase the reward value of action plans.

The fifth stage of counseling is continually to follow up the attempts of counselees to change. Even when people have terminated the counseling, the counselor must be willing to follow them and see how they are getting along.

STAGES OF FAMILY COUNSELING DURING TRANSITIONS

Assessment

Unlike traditional family therapy in which the counselor might have eight to twenty weeks of extended contact with a family, when you counsel people with unplanned pregnancies, you will probably have only two or three intensive contacts. But if you are their pastor, friend, or a family member, you might have a long period to follow up on the counseling. If your relationship with them is more casual or more formal, you might never see them again.

Because there is little time for giving help, assessment must be done quickly. In marriage counseling, I usually use three weeks to assess the couple's relationship thoroughly. In family counseling for unplanned pregnancy, I assess as I am finding out about the problem and my assessment centers around the three key variables: how much their time schedules have been disrupted, how many disagreements they must resolve, and whether the family is engaged in ongoing power struggles. I also try to find whether other life transitions are occurring simultaneously with the unplanned pregnancy.

I make other assessments as they appear appropriate, such as how depressed a woman might be or whether there is any threat of suicide or violence in the family or threats to the supposed father.

Generally, I am interested in the position of family members spiritually, because I need to gauge how to approach the family in a way that they can hear what I have to say to them. I want to frame my suggestions to each family member in ways to elicit cooperation rather than resistance.

Helping Them Understand What's Happening

As the story unfolds and I make my assessments mentally, I try to help the family understand their reactions. I might explain to them about the normal progression of crises—shock, panic, turmoil and indecision, reorganization, continued adjustment, and resolution at some different level of functioning. I will probably use the Double ABCX model of family stress to inform my thinking. I might also reflect on how the pregnancy has caused them to rearrange their activities and how it has thus disturbed their balance of intimacy and distance.

I will inquire about the frequency of conflict and describe how new decisions will inevitably result in some anger at family members. I usually do not frame instability in power structures as "power struggles" to family members. When I observe power struggles, I keep that to myself and try to help the family change their interactions so that the power struggle will be lessened. In the past, whenever I have casually remarked, "It seems as if you are in a power struggle," every eye in the room instantly fixes on me and the family members, almost in unison, say, "We are *not* in a power struggle. We are merely discussing the issues." They then turn toward each other and immediately resume their power struggles. I usually console myself in those instances by thinking how I at least unified them on one issue—putting me in my place.

As you read the above, it might seem that I am holding an intellectual seminar, dispassionately informing the family about an academic topic while they whip out their notebooks and eagerly take notes. That is, of course, not what is happening. I almost never *tell* the family something unless they have already given concrete examples from their own description. Further, I try to keep my "explanations" relatively short. Two or three sentences at the most. Even when the family asks a tempting question, such as "How *should* we deal with Karen (the pregnant teen)?" I try to make my answers and explanations short rather than elaborate. For a university professor, that is often not easy. At times I have to imagine physically being gagged to limit my talking. I know that the counseling room is rarely the place for a sermon or lecture.

Helping Change Time Schedules

If the family members' time schedules have been disrupted, you can help them change their interactions by two fundamental interventions. You might explain the difficulty and ask how they might rearrange their schedules to be more pleasing to everyone. With families involved in power struggles, however, this merely provides another arena for battle. In those instances, you can make assignments for the family to accomplish certain tasks. For example, if you detect that intimacy has been greatly reduced between the mother and father as a result of a new birth, you might suggest that the couple set aside an evening and plan how they are going to divide caretaking responsibilities for the infant. Or you might recommend that they need to get a baby-sitter and go out to eat or to the movies together. If baby-sitters are not acceptable for the couple, you might recommend that they purchase steaks (or Hamburger Helper) at the store and spend an evening preparing and eating a special meal together. Instead of going to the movies, the couple might rent a video recorder and bring movies home. Many families may not have the financial resources even to survive; yet they can think of ways to spend time that will promote closer family ties.

Generally, by making suggestions, you can short-circuit power struggles because one spouse does not have to accede to the suggestion of the other one. Even if they resist your suggestion, at least they are agreeing on something—resisting you.

Helping Manage Conflict

Decisions must be made when unplanned pregnancies occur. If the family has many disagreements, feelings might run high. You might adopt many roles in helping the family resolve their conflicts. My preference is to make the minimum possible intervention. If the family can solve their difficulties without my assistance, then I am eager to let them. I tend to be uncomfortable when strong anger is expressed, but I have come to understand that not everyone shares my discomfort. By this criterion, some families must *really* care. One family that I saw at my office cared so much that people in the building next door would ask how they were doing.

If the family is not able to resolve its differences without my intervention, then I might provide information about resolving differences. Usually, I recommend that the family buy the book, *Getting to Yes: Negotiating Agreement Without Giving In.*[11] The premise of the book is that people fail to resolve disagreements because they stake out *positions* and are unwilling to give up their positions. *Getting to Yes* involves, rather, identifying the *interests* behind the positions, then trying to think of ways that both people's interests can be met. Learning to do this requires some skill (and usually coaching from the counselor), but it is easily understood by most people. I use the book by recommending that the family members sit together and read the book aloud to each other (assuming the children are old enough to understand and have patience with the reading). Not only does this insure that the book gets read, it also provides a coactive if not intimate family experience.

If the family cannot resolve their differences with information, I might serve as referee. Or I might even mediate the discussion. My "big gun" is usually to videotape or audiotape the arguments (remember to call them "discussions" when speaking to the family) and use the tapes to give feedback about how to resolve differences more productively.

Helping Make Power Structures More Stable

Usually, little can be done in two or three meetings to change power structures, for continual power struggles are usually well-entrenched patterns of behavior that are highly resistant to change. Crises, though, can effectively disrupt power struggles as well as exacerbate them. Sometimes merely making changes in time schedules can change patterns of argument that have persisted for years. Negotiating agreement on new issues brought about by a transition can rearrange patterns of power and control, too—especially if you are able to teach the family new ways to resolve their differences.

Overall, though, I am relatively pessimistic about making large changes in long-lasting power struggles through a brief intervention. I generally aim both for helping a family solve the problems they present and for having a good experience with counseling. After that, I might recommend that they seek additional longer term counseling to resolve some of the differences that have persisted for years. Despite my pessimism, I might still try to change power struggles, usually by either changing the physical arrangement of the family members within the session or by making assignments that force the family to interact differently outside of the counseling session.

In one example, I used a Minuchin-like maneuver in which physical space became a picture of the psychological interaction. A mother and father were stubbornly disagreeing over how much to cuddle their new baby. I stood up and said, "You are both dug in to your positions so deeply that you cannot face what the other has to say. Turn your chairs back to back. That's right. Get up and turn your chairs around. Good. Now, you can continue to talk to each other."

The couple objected, "This is silly."

"It may be silly," I replied, "but it is what you have been doing. Furthermore, you have put the baby between you. Here." I jerked another chair between them and placed a sweater on it. "In your desire to get your way, you each are trying to pull the baby over to your side. That's a pretty fragile baby. I hope you don't tear it apart." That dramatic event showed that the real casualty in their continued struggles might be their child.

Another example of changing power struggles occurred with a counselor I was supervising, Tim Tehan. A family constantly argued over the discipline of their eight-year-old girl. The girl was the mother's child by a previous marriage. The mother could not control the girl, but when the father tried to discipline the girl, the mother stepped in and criticized him for being too harsh. The father withdrew. The mother would again try to discipline the child, fail, and cry to the father. The father would discipline harshly. The mother would correct, and the cycle would continue. This clever family had entertained themselves for years with this pattern.

Our plan was ultimately to get the mother and father to work together on their attempts at discipline, but it is difficult to move from one stable position to another stable position without passing through an unstable position first. We therefore defined the father as the expert on the behavior problem that the girl was having—doing chores around the house. The family agreed that the mother was the neater of the two parents, so we said that the father must better understand the difficulty that the child was having trying to pick up her things. (If the father had been neater, we probably would have said that *because* he was the neater, he was the expert.) The point was to make it easier for the father to interact with the daughter. We assigned the family the task of setting aside ten minutes each night for the father to talk pleasantly and positively about all the things that the daughter had done during the day. Criticism was strictly forbidden. The mother acted as time keeper. After trying this within the session, the mother found that she had difficulty staying out of the discussion between father and daughter. *She* suggested that she had better leave the room while the father and daughter were talking. This Haley-like strategic intervention—ten minutes of talk each day, for five days of the week (we were easy on them)—helped change the entire pattern of family interactions.

Referral

Most of us would like to believe that we can help anyone, yet our experience has shown us differently. In some cases, counseling families with unplanned pregnancies involves information or skills that we do not have. In those instances, we need to admit our limitations and refer our clients to someone who can help. One difficult struggle of the pastor and professional mental health worker is maintaining a referral list of people in whom we have confidence. Such a list can be built through networking with other pastors and professionals in the area. In addition, even after referring a family, you will want to check back with them to see how their counseling went with the other professional. Some of the professionals to whom I have referred have received poor reports from clients, which has helped me refine my referral list.

When making a referral, I usually explain to the family that I do not think that I will be able to give them the help that they need. I generally suggest the names of several potential counselors. I describe the strengths of each counselor and the location of each. Because I do not refer to counselors in whom I have no confidence, I usually do not have to worry about counselors' weaknesses. Depending on the clients, I might offer to make the initial call for them once they have decided on whom to contact, or I might simply give the clients the name and phone number of the professional and allow them to initiate the contact themselves.

Recognizing our limitations as counselors seems to occur in stages. Early in our counseling career, we may have little confidence. In the middle of our career, we might be overconfident. As we encounter failures, though, we begin to learn the types of problems and the sorts of clients with whom we work most effectively.

Termination of Counseling Sessions

Because counseling with problem pregnancies is generally short-term counseling, termination is not usually the problem it is with on-going counseling. The strong emotions of a crisis can create strong emotional bonds between you and your clients. Usually clients can be moved rapidly to independent action through treating them as responsible people throughout your contacts with them.

PART TWO

PREGNANCIES THAT ARE
TOO EARLY

CHAPTER FOUR

TEENAGE PREGNANCY

In 1976, THE ALAN GUTTMACHER INSTITUTE, which is the research organization for Planned Parenthood, described teenage pregnancy as an epidemic in their publication, *11 Million Teenagers: What Can Be Done About the Epidemic of Adolescent Pregnancy in the United States?*[1] Although there was some evidence that the rate of pregnancies to adolescents had decreased linearly from the late 1950s (about 95 live births per 1000 adolescents between ages 15 and 19) to about 1970 (about 68 live births per 1000 adolescents between ages 15 and 19), we are indebted to the Guttmacher Institute for raising the conscience of the nation about the sexual performance of our youth.

Statistics cannot capture the heartache of the millions of teen pregnancies that have been unplanned in recent decades. Nor can statistics reveal the horror of the millions of aborted babies in those years. But statistics can show that the local congregation—even if small—has a good chance of having a family or several families with unplanned teenage pregnancies.

In 1983, the number of births to teens under twenty was 499,038—14 percent of all births.[2] Most of those births were unintended. Most births to teens were to older teens. In 1983, there were 9,752 births to girls under 15, while there were 172,673 to girls 15 through 17, and 316,613 to girls 18 and 19. Total births were down from similar statistics in 1960 and 1970 (see Table 1).

Statistics about frequency of live births to adolescents tell only half the story. Since *Roe* v. *Wade* (January 22, 1973), abortions have soared. In 1973, 23 abortions per 1000 women were reported in young women ages 15 to 19. In 1980, almost 43 abortions per 1000 women were reported. The rate of total pregnancies per thousand 15 to 19-year-olds has steadily increased since *Roe* v. *Wade*, from 83 in 1973 to 96 in 1980.

Births to Adolescents According to Age of the Mother (U.S.A.)				
Age	1960	1970	1980	1983
Under 15	7,462	11,752	10,169	9,752
15-17	177,904	223,590	198,222	172,673
18-19	423,775	421,118	353,939	316,613
Total	609,141	656,460	562,330	499,038

Table 1

TWO TRAGEDIES

Rhonda

Rhonda was a cheerleader and president of the junior class at her high school when she discovered that she was pregnant. The father of the child was her boyfriend since the eighth grade. She said that they had just drifted into sex as they continued to date. Their love had grown and they had intercourse in the summer before their junior year in high school during a weekend that Tim spent at the lake with Rhonda. Since then, lovemaking had become increasingly frequent until it took place almost every weekend at least once. Tim had taken responsibility for birth control, using the condom, but the method was (obviously) not foolproof.

Rhonda and her family were involved in early discussions about the pregnancy. Their Catholic beliefs were largely responsible for never considering abortion. Tim also told his family, and the two families had a conference. During that time, Rhonda and Tim announced their plans to marry. The parents were cautiously accepting of the decision because they wanted a legitimate solution for the problem.

After marriage, Rhonda and Tim decided that Tim would finish high school but Rhonda would raise the child. She would finish high school later, they decided. Tim completed high school with little difficulty but was able to find only low-paying work after graduating. Instead of finishing high school, Rhonda went to work to supplement Tim's low income. The strains of child rearing and financial difficulties provided a catalyst for resentment about the forced marriage to flourish. After four years, Rhonda and Tim separated, divorcing the following year. Rhonda finally got her G.E.D. after Jennifer, the child, graduated from high school herself.

Sharon

Fourteen-year-old Sharon came to the Crisis Pregnancy Center because she had missed a period and was afraid that she might be pregnant. After the pregnancy test, the counselor confirmed her worst fears. Being a Christian, Sharon wanted to do what was right. She decided that she would have the baby. The counselor at the center convinced Sharon that she should tell her parents about her pregnancy.

The next morning Sharon and her parents were back at the center demanding to see the counselor. Sharon's eyes were red from crying. Her father led the conversation by saying, "You have to talk some sense into Sharon. She's pregnant and she refuses to have an abortion. If she doesn't terminate this pregnancy, it will be a millstone around her neck for the rest of her life. A child of a fourteen-year-old will ruin Sharon's childhood. She'll have to worry about the child when she should be having fun in high school. She'll have financial pressures all her life. She'll be dumping the kid on her mother and me all the time. *You* tell her," he said to the counselor, "that what I'm saying is true. Tell her that if she has an abortion, it'll all be over and she can forget about this horrible nightmare."

"Mr. Merle," said the counselor, "I'd really like to hear what your wife thinks about this."

"He's right," said Mrs. Merle. "When I was a teenager, I became pregnant. Our first son, Mike, was born when Charles and I were only seventeen. Of course, we got married before the birth. But now, I see how immature we were. We weren't really able to raise Mike like we should have. We made lots of mistakes with him that we didn't make with the other two. I've often wished I had been able to have an abortion. And it's worse for Sharon. She's only fourteen—nowhere near ready for marriage. She says that she and the boy have no intention to marry. It'll ruin her life if she has that child. The abortion is so easy and quick. I want you to talk her into it."

"How about you, Sharon?" said the counselor. "What is your thinking?"

"Well, I still. . . ."

"Wait a minute," interrupted her father. "It is really irrelevant what she thinks. She is still a minor, and her mother and I will decide what she is going to do about this pregnancy."

"Mr. Merle," said the counselor. "I am sure that you and Mrs. Merle want to do what is best for Sharon and that you don't just want to impose a solution on her. In fact, my bet is that your openness is why you came with her here this morning rather than dragging her off to an abortion clinic. You *want* her to be happy and involved with the decision. Am I reading you correctly?"

"Yes, that's right. We did come here because we wanted Sharon to agree with our decision."

"Let's allow Sharon to tell about her feelings. She talked with me at some length yesterday, and she seemed to use very mature reasoning in coming to her decision about what to do with her baby. Did she explain her decision to you?"

"She told us she wanted to have the baby," said Mrs. Merle, "but that wouldn't be right. Not at her age."

"It would, too, be right," Sharon broke in. "What you want to do is not right. You want to murder my baby."

"Now just a minute . . ." began Mr. Merle.

"Hold it a minute, Sharon," said the counselor. "Yesterday, you discussed this calmly. Do you think you can do that today?"

"Okay."

Sharon then described her beliefs that the baby was a life that God had given her to care for while it was within her body. She said that it was not hers to do with as she wanted. Rather, it was a gift that she was holding for someone else. It was God's child. She used an analogy that she said she had heard from her Sunday School teacher, Karen.

"It's like I was given a precious diamond to hold," she began. "Then, as I was looking at it, a thief broke in and started to hold everyone up. When the thief wasn't looking, I might swallow the diamond so the thief couldn't get it. But then the next day the owner of the diamond might come to me and say, 'Thank you for saving my precious diamond. I'll pay you a reward when you return it.' But I might say, 'What do you mean return it? It's part of my body. I can do whatever I want with it.' You see, Mom and Dad, I'm just holding God's child for him. I can't decide just to kill it."

Sharon and her parents continued to discuss the decision for two and one-half hours. When they left, the counselor felt that they understood each other more, even though they did not agree. Six months later, the counselor saw Sharon in a large shopping mall. She was not pregnant.

The counselor approached Sharon and initiated a conversation. Repentant, Sharon explained that her parents had kept constant pressure on her for about two weeks, threatening her with force and with withdrawal of love. Finally, she relented. Since then, she felt overwhelmed with guilt for giving in.

As sad as this tale is, it is not finished. Three months after the meeting at the mall, Sharon again came to the Crisis Pregnancy Center. Pregnant. This time, she said, she was determined to care for God's child in the proper way.

WHAT IS AN ADOLESCENT?

An adolescent is a person between the onset of puberty through the end of the teen years. Although there is no clearly agreed upon way to categorize adolescents, the period is generally divided into early adolescence (10–14), middle adolescence (15–17), and late adolescence (18–19). For girls, menarche begins with the onset of menses between eight and sixteen. The mean age of the onset of menarche is about twelve—a little earlier for black girls and a little later for white girls. Ovulation usually occurs within two years after the onset of menarche, so that over 95 percent of all girls are fully capable of childbearing by 18. For boys, the average age of their first nocturnal emission is about twelve also.

One misleading aspect of research on teen pregnancies is that differentiation among adolescents according to age has not been made consistently. As we saw earlier, the birth rate for girls fifteen through seventeen was forty times as great as the birth rate for early adolescents. The birth rate for late adolescent girls was about 135 times as great as for the early adolescent and about four times as great as the middle adolescent. Furthermore, the percent of births born out of wedlock shows even greater differentials.

Adolescent pregnancy is an occasion for multiple decisions. Adults think of decisions as logical and rational, but adolescents make decisions for many other reasons. To understand the thinking of adolescents, four concepts are necessary: (a) the cognitive development of the adolescent, (b) the moral development of the adolescent, (c) the importance of the way that the adolescent defines sexuality decisions, and (d) the role of the family in the values of the adolescent.

Cognitive Development of Adolescents

According to Piaget,[3] adolescence is a time when the child moves from the cognitive stage of concrete operations to the stage of formal operations. *Operations* means the ability to manipulate objects mentally. The manipulation is motivated by *equilibration,* which means resolving a tension between the environment and the person's mental or physical capabilities.

Equilibration can occur through *assimilation* or *accommodation*. Assimilation means that the person handles information that does not fit comfortably into his or her current understanding by distorting the information so that it fits current understanding. Accommodation means that the person handles information that does not fit his or her current understanding by changing that understanding to accurately interpret the environment.

Piaget found that cognitive ability developed regularly through four stages. Although there is some controversy about the exact age at which people reach each stage,[4] most cognitive psychologists who have tested Piaget's theory believe that the stages occur in regular order and that people move gradually rather than precipitously from one stage to another. This is especially true of the move to the most mature stage, formal operations. The four stages of cognitive development, according to Piaget, are sensori-motor (0–2 years), preoperational (2–7 years), concrete operational (7–11 years), and formal operational (12–adult years). The ages in parentheses refer to the onset of capabilities to think with the maturity of that stage.

Adolescents' thinking is mostly characterized by a mixture of concrete operational thinking and formal operational thinking. During early adolescence most of the thinking is concrete operational thinking with formal operational thinking only occurring in fits and starts. In middle adolescence, there is an unpredictable mixture of concrete and formal operational thinking. By late adolescence, thinking of the adolescent is mostly formal operational.

Concrete operational thinking is largely characteristic of early and middle adolescents. Concrete operations involve thinking about specific objects and events rather than about abstract ideas. Much of the time, early (and to a lesser extent middle) adolescents have difficulty anticipating future outcomes and logically and systematically solving problems. Rather than examining all the available alternatives, early and middle adolescents are likely to be influenced by specific situational pressures. Because early adolescents' thinking is not fully systematic, they probably will not understand complex effects. In other words, they may understand how this pregnancy affects them personally but not even think how it affects their parents, their siblings, or others.

Concrete operational thinking can greatly affect the way an early or middle adolescent girl makes decisions about her sexual behavior. For example, when given sex information not in line with her expectations, an early adolescent girl might merely assimilate the information so that it fits with her preexisting beliefs. A sex education teacher might assume that if an early adolescent girl is given accurate biological information about reproduction, she will change her ideas about how daring and how much fun intercourse is, tempering her desires by understanding the consequences of pregnancy. The early or middle adolescent, though, might assimilate the sex information within her already existing beliefs. Instead of reasoning, "If I have sex, I might get pregnant and it would be devastating," the early adolescent might think, "If I have sex, there is only a very small chance I'll get pregnant." This is complicated by the "egocentricism" of the typical adolescent.[5] This egocentricism results in a "personal fable." "Sure, there is a small chance I'll get pregnant," she might think, "but it'll never happen to *me*. I can't get pregnant. I won't get sexually transmitted disease" (STD). Rather than accommodate (change) her beliefs to the reality of possible pregnancy, the early or middle adolescent will likely assimilate the information to justify her behavior.

In addition to using assimilation when the adult might expect her to use accommodation, the early or middle adolescent might be overly responsive to immediate concrete situations—such as a boy pressuring her to have sex or her sexual arousal or her curiosity or a "soap opera" she is watching on afternoon television before her parents get home from work. She might fail to see the many things that can happen in the future as a result of the act of sex. In periods of reflection, she might be able to see that pregnancy would have a large impact on her *own* life, but she cannot see the enormous impact the pregnancy might have on her family. In fact, she probably would not consider her family in her deliberations except to think about how angry or disappointed they might be in her. The effect of her pregnancy on their lives would probably never be considered.

Thus, the early and middle adolescent might not only choose to make an illogical decision about whether to have sex, the early and middle adolescent might *not even be capable of* making a logical decision that considers all the alternatives carefully and arrives at a sound conclusion. This is especially true in an emotionally charged situation.

Although I used the decision about whether to have sex with a boy as an example of decision-making restrictions on the adolescent in her low teens, the same restrictions might apply to any decision required of the pregnant adolescent. The impact of abortion, the decision to bear the child to term and raise him or her, and the decision to place the child for adoption might all be clouded by concrete thinking.

Moral Development of Adolescents

Limited by her ability to make logical decisions by formal operational thinking, the early and middle adolescent uses other methods to make decisions. One possible tool is moral reasoning. Kohlberg[6] has identified six "universal" stages through which he claims moral reasoning develops. Snarey[7] has provided some support for the claims that Kohlberg's stages of moral reasoning are universal, though there are still unanswered methodological questions about the research.

In the most basic stage of moral development, the child reasons that "might makes right." Generally, fear of punishment controls the actions of the child. In the second stage, the person is controlled by the desire for pleasure. The third stage is characterized by acceptance of the values of respected people. If peers, parents, school teachers, or counselors recommend a course of action, the adolescent is likely to go along with the recommendation of the most respected people. In the fourth stage, law controls moral decisions. There is an appreciation that laws must be obeyed, so the adolescent obeys. In the fifth stage, the adolescent reasons that laws are social contracts and that one's responsibility to other people in society is the final arbiter of moral action. In the sixth stage of moral development, the adolescent reasons that transcendent higher truths control moral action.

Generally, adolescents will reason using the lower stages of

Kohlberg's scheme. They might go along with parents' or other authority figures' desires because they perceive them as powerful—much as Sharon did with her parents. Or they might be governed by their desires, simply having sex because it is pleasurable or electing abortion because it is more convenient than giving birth to the child. Or they might be pressured by peers or parents or teachers to have sex or to have an abortion or to raise the child or to place the child for adoption. In each case social acceptance is the motivating force. Or the adolescent might use law to justify his or her actions—reasoning that adolescents have a right to contraceptives (*Carey* v. *Population Services International,* 1977) or that adolescents have the right to abortion (*Roe* v. *Wade*); so, if it is legally right, then it must be personally right.[8]

Whatever the stage of moral reasoning they are in, adolescents (like adults) can use their moral reasoning ability to justify whatever they want to do. The counselor, though, must assess the stage of moral development of the adolescent in order to know how to talk with the girl or boy in a way that she or he can understand.

Morality or Lifestyle? How Sexual Decisions Are Defined

Just because an adult might view the decision to engage in sexual intercourse outside of marriage as a moral decision does not mean an adolescent will define it that way. Peers, school systems, and much of the popular media have portrayed sex outside of marriage *not* as a moral decision but as a *lifestyle* decision. Peers of adolescents, motivated to determine their sexual identity,[9] want to engage in sexual acts to establish themselves as adults. School systems, sensitive to the charge that they are promoting religious or moral values, have defined sexual decisions as amoral lifestyle decisions, or, at best, moral decisions that depend on each individual's moral standards. Media, motivated by profit, portray sex as a marketable commodity, using it to promote products, to convey story lines, and to achieve an "R" rating. Adolescents generally report that most of the specific information they have about sex comes from peers and the media.[10] Both sources of information frame the issue as a lifestyle issue rather than a moral issue.

When sex is conceptualized by adolescents as a moral issue, different thoughts are stimulated than when sex is conceptualized as a lifestyle issue. Recall that early and middle adolescents often do not reason systematically and abstractly in emotion-charged situations. When they discuss sex with their peers or in the classroom, they often think according to what they see before them. They might argue for freedom of choice in sexual conduct, proabortion, and for libertarian values. In a weekend discussion at Sunday school or that evening with their parents, the same adolescents might argue for chastity, prolife, and conservative values. Are they two-faced or, worse, lying to someone? Not necessarily. They might simply be incapable of bringing the arguments together into a rational resolution. For such adolescents, the way they define the situation—moral or lifestyle—will govern their behavior.

The counselor must realize that an early or middle adolescent will tend to think about his or her decision differently depending on whose presence he or she is in. The wise counselor will ask the adolescent to imagine talking with a boyfriend or girlfriend, peers, parents, and other significant people. Help him or her define the problem as a moral dilemma regardless of who the adolescent might talk to. Then help them marshall arguments before being exposed to other people in real-life encounters.

ADOLESCENT-FAMILY RELATIONSHIPS

Is There Hope for Moral Adolescents?

The typical adolescent spends most of the day at school and with friends. For parents concerned about the moral decisions of their child, this can sound discouraging. Parents will undoubtedly lose influence over their children because they cannot control the situations they encounter. Can parents hope that adolescents will adopt the parents' values during adolescence when most adolescents—especially middle to late adolescents—are forging their own values from their backgrounds and current surroundings? Yes, there is hope.

81

Clark and Worthington[11] have reviewed empirical research on the transmission of religious values from parents to adolescents. They concluded that adolescents are strongly affected by the values of their parents. Mothers and fathers may both be influential, depending on how much time they spend with daughters or sons. The prominence of the value within the home is crucial in determining the degree to which an adolescent adopts the parents' values. Beliefs are more easily adopted than the devotional practices of parents. Furthermore, perceptions of the adolescents about their parents' values are more influential than the parents' actual values.

Several family characteristics affect the degree to which the adolescent will adopt the parents' values. Family conflict, which is common in families of adolescents, affects transmission of religious values. High degrees of conflict inhibit adolescents' adoption of their parents' values despite whether the conflict is between the parents or between one or more of the parents and the adolescent. Intimacy within the family can also promote transmission of values from parents to adolescents. Warm families share values more often than distant families. Finally, parents who are characterized by high degrees of parental support and control are more likely to have adolescents whose values are similar to their own than are other families. These findings are especially true in early adolescence but become less certain as the child passes from middle to late adolescence.

Pubertal Status

Thus, the influence of parents depends on a number of family characteristics. The adolescent's pubertal status is also important. As the child becomes an adolescent, family interactions change. For example, boys gain power within the family at the expense of the mother as they pass through puberty. At the onset of puberty, boys begin to interrupt parents more. Mothers, even those who carefully explained each decision prior to the onset of puberty, begin to give their early adolescent sons commands without also supplying reasons. This provokes conflict between the boy and the mother. Usually the father will act as the peacemaker during periods of conflict.

As the boy matures, the mother asserts herself less, and the boy gets his way more often. The exchange of power has generally flowed from the mother to the son with the father's power being little affected.[12]

The pubertal girl usually gains power at the expense of the father.[13] Usually the beginning of the development of breasts signals the change in family interactions. The father and daughter, who previously had conversed in straight on, open postures, tend to turn slightly askew after breast development begins. Their interaction resembles two adults talking more than a parent-child conversation. Fathers tend to treat their girl adolescents more like adults, deferring to their wishes more after puberty than before puberty.

Role of Family Prior to Adolescent Pregnancy

Problems with teenage sexuality can arise within the family whenever parents fail to give the adolescent additional power beyond childhood status. Usually, adolescence is a time of the gradual transfer of power in which the child tries to pull power from parents while parents try to restrain the child.

Generally, problem pregnancies have been associated with a number of these family patterns. Pannor *et al.*[14] have found that adolescent girls who have become pregnant generally perceive their lives characterized by repeated conflict, within the family or with the outside world. The *perception* of conflict was more important than the presence of observable conflict. Abernathy[15] found that the adolescent's perception of the mother-daughter relationship as problematic was a predictor of adolescent pregnancy. Nor was mother-daughter conflict the only important conflict. Perry and Millemit[16] found that families characterized by rule instability, disagreement, conflict, and criticism were associated with problem pregnancies. Others have found that pregnant adolescents often were from homes in which one parent was dead or absent through separation or divorce.[17] Cheetham found that fathers of pregnant adolescents were often domineering and cruel.[18] Meyerowitz and Maler found high incidence of adolescent pregnancy in girls who felt social rejection, hopelessness, loss of control, and apathy. Other less predictive characteristics were a desire to leave home and passive response to aggression.[19] Fisher and Scharf also found that girls who became pregnant generally were either trying to resolve parent-child conflicts or to simply find a way out of a conflict-ridden home.[20]

The picture that emerges from the various studies of adolescent pregnancy in the family is that families that are loving, warm, and that have infrequent conflict and criticism generally transmit their values accurately to their adolescents; whereas families that are in conflict, critical, and judgmental often have adolescents who act out sexually and become pregnant.

Conflict between mother and father can stimulate the girl to have a "problem" in the hope that it will divert parents from their own conflict.[21] By sacrificing herself, the adolescent hopes to protect her parents from divorce.

When the conflict is between parents and the adolescent, other causes are generally at work. Some researchers have suggested that sexual acting out by a teenage girl is one way to assert power so that parents cannot control her.[22] Stierlin found that rejecting parents push some girls into crisis runaway situations.[23]

Vincent found five differences between pregnant and nonpregnant adolescent girls from families of lower socioeconomic status.[24] Pregnant adolescent girls generally came from families with minimal parental discipline and were given decision-making freedom early in their lives. The girls, bereft of parental guidance, turned to peers, identifying strongly with them. They reported peers to be more influential than their parents. Finally, pregnant adolescent girls had minimal exposure to the church or conventional values about sexual behavior. Despite finding these discriminators, Vincent concluded that there was no single constellation of family variables that predicted pregnancy in adolescence. He found that girls from many types of families become pregnant. This finding was echoed a quarter of a century later by the Group for the Advancement of Psychiatry, who reviewed the research on teen pregnancy.[25]

Pannor studied middle socioeconomic-class girls who were pregnant and others who were not pregnant. Pregnant girls appeared to be motivated by self-pleasure and personal gain, while others' needs were not prominent in their thinking.[26]

Furstenberg (1976) identified three reasons why girls engage in sexual activity.[27] Most commonly, girls cited a perceived inability to resist peer pressure. Other girls cited emotional involvement with their partner and failure to see any good reason for waiting. Rains[28] identified emotional involvement with a partner as a strategy pursued by middle-class adolescents to neutralize guilt and fear over acting against parent-advocated mores. Generally, teens in middle-class socioeconomic groups allow "love" to grow gradually. It proceeds in gradual stages from the perception of love to monogamous dating to increased sexual participation to maintenance of technical virginity to a "spontaneous" lovemaking episode to the regular use or nonuse of contraceptives. Usually the spontaneous lovemaking episode is characterized by invoking the "personal fable"[29]—it'll never happen to *me*.

Role of Family Post-Pregnancy

Once the adolescent becomes pregnant, the family is involved in decisions. In well over half the instances, pregnant teens involve at least their mothers in their decision between abortion or bearing to term.[30] Generally, the pregnant adolescent, having just discovered her pregnancy, is reluctant to involve the family. The usual parental response to finding out their daughter is pregnant is anger. Often the anger is mixed with shame and guilt.[31] The announcement of pregnancy is often perceived as a symbol of failure for the morals and aspirations of the entire family.

Girls accurately fear the anger that will be provoked. Often the girl will want to have a pastor or counselor present when she tells her family. The family, being angry and ashamed of the pregnancy, will often react with some hostility to the idea of meeting with a counselor or pastor. The beginning of such counseling will be laced with defensiveness and the counselor must work especially hard to diffuse the sense of guilt and judgment that the family feels. Ultimately, the family and the girl will accept the child.[32] For example, Bowerman *et al.*[33] found that two-thirds of the white respondents and four-fifths of their black respondents believed that the infant of the pregnant adolescent belonged to the entire family.

Just because families come to accept the child does not mean that there was not turmoil after the discovery of the pregnancy. Bernstein recounted that adolescents who elect to bear the child to term and who live in the house of their parents during the pregnancy have family interactions characterized by stress and confusion throughout most of the pregnancy, and in some cases even beyond the birth of the child.[34]

Just as there is no single way to predict which adolescent girls will become pregnant, there is no single family response to pregnancy. Four possibilities exist, but each family response is unique. First, families which were supportive of the adolescent before pregnancy continue to provide necessary support after the pregnancy is discovered. Necessary support involves (a) caring acceptance, (b) help with physical and monetary needs, (c) help solving problems, and (d) help with personal maturity. Second, some families that provided support prior to the pregnancy become disorganized with the announcement of the pregnancy and blame the girl. They generally experience much turmoil soon after the pregnancy is discovered. Some will pull together in a "honeymoon" period and outwardly support the girl while giving subtle messages of blame.[35] Others will be openly critical of the girl throughout her pregnancy. Third, some families that were unsupportive prior to the pregnancy may be galvanized by the crisis and bond together to form a cohesive, supportive unit. Fourth, other families that were unsupportive prior to the pregnancy will continue to devalue the girl after the pregnancy is discovered.

Role of Family Post-Delivery

Generally, a number of options are possible after the birth of the child. For instance, the mother may place the child for adoption through public channels—in which case the mother relinquishes all rights to see the child again—or through private adoption channels—in which case the mother might work out a number of arrangements about seeing the child and meeting his or her adoptive parents. Adoption occurs only about 5 percent of the time. Second, the mother may be uncertain about whether to place the child for adoption. She might place the child in a professional foster home until the decision about adoption or child rearing can be made. Third, the mother might decide to keep the child and raise it herself. This is by far the most common option.[36] A number of options are possible here, too. The mother may marry the father of the child, and they might either live in their parents' household, which happens about two-thirds of the time,[37] or they might establish their own household. Or the mother might elect to remain a single parent, which is gaining social acceptability.[38] If the mother raises the child as a single parent, then the mother might establish her own household or might live with her parents. Her parents—usually her mother—might be involved greatly or not at all. Usually, the adolescent mother is the primary care giver, but occasionally turns the child over to the grandmother.[39] In many families, though, childrearing responsibilities are diffused among all the members in the household.[40] The willingness of the adolescent to establish her own household and to assume primary caregiving responsibility for the infant depends on the age of the adolescent and her family environment.

Volumes of research have summarized the childrearing abilities and skills of the adolescent mother. Most researchers agree that the level of parenting skill shown by adolescent mothers is not high. However, after a thorough review of the empirical literature, Roosa *et al.* concluded that most of the knowledge about the skill level of teenage mothers "is based on myth rather than empirical fact."[41] They cited poor socioeconomic status, family support systems, marital stability, nutrition, and prenatal care as possibly being more important than adolescent status of the mother in predicting poor mothering skills.

Regardless of their actual level of competence as mothers, though, most adolescent mothers do not feel *prepared* to be mothers. Girls under fifteen predictably feel the least prepared to function as mothers. Furstenberg[42] found that two-thirds of the mothers under fifteen were openly hostile to being a parent and felt unable to be a good parent. At seventeen or older, 45 percent of the adolescent mothers felt hostile toward motherhood and unable to handle the responsibilities. On the other hand, the same groups later were found to be equally capable mothers and to have equally good relationships with their children.

If the adolescent maintains close ties with her family of origin, especially if she lives with them after the birth, the teen's mother will generally be involved to some extent in child rearing.[43] Most likely, the adolescent's mother will not play the role of the typical grandmother. The adolescent's mother (and father) must help the adolescent function as an effective adolescent with a social life that provides opportunities for her to mature relatively normally while simultaneously helping the adolescent to learn parenting skills and responsibilities. At the same time, the parents of the adolescent must continue to support and nurture her as she copes with the additional duties of motherhood and with the social stigma of being an unwed mother.

If the adolescent marries, the newlyweds will often live near one or both sets of parents. Adjusting to marriage and parenthood simultaneously places a great strain on the relationship, which results in an extremely high rate of divorce. For example, Furstenberg found that 20 percent of adolescent mothers who married divorced within one year of marriage; 33 percent divorced within two years; 50 percent within four years; and 60 percent within six years of marriage.[44] The families of the adolescent parents will be strongly tempted to be heavily involved in the lives of their children if the relationships between the adolescents and their parents are at all positive. This can exacerbate power struggles between married adolescents who are trying to work out the rules of their relationship.

Because the relationship between adolescent parents is more than likely to be troubled, the counselor who sees the couple for counseling might be tempted to work on the marriage relationship and to ignore some of the more mundane elements of the marriage such as problems of financial support and employment difficulties.[45] The counselor must remain alert to parenting skills, basic survival necessities, and relationships with the maternal and paternal grandparents besides attending to the marital relationship between the adolescents.

ADOLESCENT DECISION MAKING

As should be obvious by now, adolescent pregnancy is a time characterized more than any problem pregnancy described in this book by *decision making,* and generally by the people least equipped to make good decisions. In Table 2, I have listed some of the decisions that might have to be made by the adolescent who becomes pregnant.

Some Decisions Involved in Adolescent Pregnancy

Will I have sex now? (decision made in each specific situation)

Will I use contraception or will my partner use contraception or will neither of us use contraception?

When should I go for a pregnancy test? Where?

Who should I tell that I am pregnant? In what order should I tell them?

Should I have an abortion or bear the child to term?

Where should I stay during the pregnancy?

Should I place the child for adoption or raise it myself?

How much should my mother be involved in raising my child?

Should I get married?

Should I drop out of school?

Is premarital sex a moral decision or is it merely a matter of my individual choice? Who will I listen to: parents, church, peers, teachers, or date partner?

Table 2

Given this variety of decisions that might confront the adolescent girl, it is helpful to understand how she might make decisions. Imagine that we can take a metaphorical trip into the mind of an adolescent and eavesdrop on her thoughts. As we shrink, we find ourselves in the middle of a large circular room. The room is dimly lit, but by squinting, we can make out a number of closed doors. We have a flashlight, which we shine on one of the doors. Its label says "Parents." We push a button beside the doorway and the doorway slides open to reveal her mother clearly saying, "Honey, your body belongs to God. It is the temple of the Holy Spirit. You need to keep yourself pure until you are married. Save sex for marriage and you and the husband that God has picked out for you will be happier." In the background we can see her father, but the messages he gives are less clearly understood. He seems to be saying that she should save sex for marriage, but we cannot be sure exactly what his thoughts are. When we turn the flashlight away from the doorway, it slides closed noiselessly.

As we examine other doorways, we find them labeled "Peers," "Pastor," "Siblings," "Teachers," "Steady Boyfriend," and several others. We soon discover that the doorways on which we shine our light (and thus focus our attention) govern the voices we hear. Some of the doorways are bigger and more noticeable than others. Some of them, such as one with the name of a boy who seems to be out for nothing but sex for himself, are boarded shut.

As we examine the remainder of the room, we find some hallways labeled "Reward Likelihood." We see signs representing the rewards certain actions will bring. For example, when she thinks about having sex with her boyfriend, a green sign springs up which says, "Feels Good." Another green sign next to it says, "Adventure," but a red sign says, "Danger of Being Caught." Altogether, the green signs are much larger than the red one, though. In the background is another red sign. It appears very small but we realize that it seems small because it is so far in the future and because it seems so unlikely. It says, "Possible Pregnancy." Another seemingly small sign says, "Possible Sexual Disease." It is hard to focus on the red signs that are so far away because the near and bright green signs are so much more eye-catching.

Now, it is one thing to stand in the middle of this adolescent's mind and look casually around when nothing much is going on, but it is an entirely different matter when things start to happen. The girl becomes involved in a dating situation in which she is alone with her boyfriend. Suddenly, there are lights flashing all around. Noise and emotion distract us. As the lights flash around the room, the most noticeable areas are the hallways giving the immediate rewards. The flashlight which can illuminate the doorway of parents or pastor seem almost insignificant when the big laser show is underway. Generally, long-term consequences are easily dismissable by thinking, "It'll never happen to me." We also find that when she thinks, "It's okay because we're in love," the voices of her peers can be heard and blend with the lasers that focus so clearly on the immediate consequences.

In this instance, our adolescent is likely to make the decision to make love with her boyfriend if she has not taken some precautions previously. One possible precaution is to increase the size of the doorways of parents, pastors, and peers that support chastity. Another is to preplan a strategy that whenever the lights distract, she consciously turns her flashlight on the parents' door and on the long-term risks and dangers associated with premarital intercourse. Finally, another way to control the outcome is to control the lasers—that is, to interrupt the sequence of events so that they do not lead toward the emotion-charged decisions that could result in premarital pregnancy.

Although this metaphor is somewhat simplistic, it represents a combination of two cognitive theories of decision making. One theory, developed by Ainslie[46] assumes that behaviors are governed by perceived rewards and punishments. The second theory that can be applied to adolescent sexual decision making is Fishbein's[47] model. Behavior or the intention to perform a behavior depends on the adolescent's attitude toward it, beliefs about what significant others think, and her motivation to comply with the significant others. Jorgensen and Sonstegard[48] have tested Fishbein's model in predicting adolescent sexual and contraceptive behavior. They found peers' beliefs to have little power in predicting the frequency of sexual intercourse of adolescents. Rather, attitudes toward the behavior and parents' beliefs predicted adolescent intercourse decisions. None of the variables predicted the use of contraceptives.

Besides lending support for a cognitive model of decision making employed by adolescents, this research showed that the values of the parents of adolescents are important in guiding their sexual behavior.

ADVICE, ACCEPTANCE, AND ABSOLUTION

Advice

As a pastor or counselor, you will generally be called on—at least in part—to help the pregnant adolescent and her family make decisions. You can give both advice and help with decision making. Your strategy in dealing with the entire family and in dealing with the adolescent alone will likely differ. In Appendix 1 I have recommended some readings to assist the counselor, the pregnant adolescent, and her family.

When you see the adolescent alone, you will usually help her think about things that she might not have considered before. For example, she might have thought about some of the ways that the pregnancy might affect her—though the extent of her thinking depends strongly on her level of cognitive development. She will be unlikely to think about how the pregnancy might affect her parents. She will probably focus on the immediate consequences of the pregnancy. Her attention will rest on the high probability that her parents will be angry and disappointed with her because she has become pregnant. You can help her see that in time, her most helpful resource is likely to be her parents and that most parents come to accept the pregnancy and the child over a few months—especially if the family can attend counseling where family members can work out how to cope with the crisis. She will likely think of abortion as an immediate solution to the problem, especially if she consulted her friends prior to consulting you. You can help her see that the after-effects of abortion are long-lasting. Bolton has said, "The emotional problems related to having had an abortion have been described as being no greater than the emotional problems associated with childbirth and child rearing."[49] Further, Miller found that adolescents with problems before an abortion were those with the most problems after the abortion.[50]

When you see the adolescent with her family, you will be dealing both with more mature decision makers and adolescents simultaneously. The temptation is to talk with the other adults. The adolescent might find that demeaning and resist your future efforts to help. On the other hand, the mature decision-making ability of the parents might be clouded by their anger, guilt, and disappointment. They might see the pregnancy as a problem to which an immediate solution is required; thus, they might pressure you and the adolescent to decide on seemingly immediate solutions. Your task in dealing with the emotionally upset family is to calm them and help them engage their powers of rationality to where they can examine the long-term alternatives that are available.

Acceptance

When a pregnant adolescent decides to include you in her decision making and in her efforts to cope with her problem pregnancy, she is usually not merely asking for information and advice about which decisions to make and about how to make those decisions. She also wants your support and acceptance. Often, the pregnant girl will want your support as she informs her parents about her pregnancy. She has asked for your help because she believes you will be able to diffuse her parents' anger and disappointment and so that she can feel that someone is in her corner—someone that her parents are also likely to respect.

Despite your initial reaction to the girl's revelation that she is pregnant, you must accept her as a person if you are to keep the lines of communication open throughout her pregnancy. Scripturally, we know that we are each imperfect and fallen. Our status as sinners does not mean that we are unimportant or unlovable. We know that, "While we were yet sinners, Christ died for us" (Rom. 5:8b KJV). We, too, are to love the sinner, which we can do without condoning her act.

One of the areas in which it is most difficult for us to show acceptance is teenage pregnancy. It is one of the most hotly debated topics at present, and most Christians have strong feelings about the morality involved in teen pregnancy, abortion, and other issues of sexuality. It is easy to put our political hat on, so to speak, when we are confronted with a pregnant teen. We might launch into a moral lecture conditioned by our political battles and by sermons of exhortation previously preached. We can easily feel that the pregnant teen has rejected our teaching about the morality of premarital intercourse and has thereby rejected and devalued us. It is easy to respond with defensiveness, blaming, condemnation, and attack. These are the temptations that must be recognized and combatted if we are to help the girl and her family. It might make us feel self-righteous to say, "I told you so and you didn't listen." It might make us feel righteous to extort a confession from the girl on the spot. Yet, as correct as we might be, we will likely lose the girl's confidence.

Absolution

The girl's immediate need for advice and acceptance does not eliminate her need for forgiveness and absolution. Yet forgiveness follows confession and repentance. Confession is brought about in the most effective sense by the work of the Holy Spirit. Our initial job is not to be the hammer of the Holy Spirit through guilt manipulation. We are to be the vessel of the Holy Spirit for love and acceptance. We might gently raise spiritual and forgiveness issues when appropriate, but generally our most productive role is to be there when the girl is ready to confess her sins, repent, and turn from them. Then we can confidently proclaim God's forgiveness to her. If we are pastors or explicitly Christian counselors, our counselees will usually know that we stand for holiness. We rarely have to initiate self-exploration of our counselees' sins (though sometimes we do). Usually our new presence will stimulate spiritual self-examination.

INVOLVING THE FAMILY IN COUNSELING

Overall, individual counseling with pregnant adolescents has not been extremely effective. Johnson and Szurek[51] reported that their individual treatment of pregnant adolescents was characterized by broken appointments, lack of compliance with treatment recommendations, and little commitment to counseling. In two independent studies of girls receiving abortion counseling, girls who elected abortion without pressure from the counselor or other significant person were least likely to experience later negative reactions from the abortion.[52] Low found that pregnant adolescents who underwent behavioral treatment in a residential program responded differently to treatment depending on their age.[53] Younger girls benefited less from the counseling than older adolescents.

Individual Versus Family Counseling with Pregnant Adolescents

Atkinson, Winzelberg, and Holland studied forty Anglo-American and forty Mexican-American pregnant adolescents who sought individual counseling at a Planned Parenthood agency.[54] They were randomly assigned to counselors who had either the same or different ethnicity and counselors who recommended either individual counseling or family counseling for resolution of the pregnancy problems. Generally, ethnicity of the counselor was not related to the preference for counselor nor was the recommendation of the counselor for individual or family treatment predictive of preference of counselor. Overall, Mexican-American girls were more trusting of their counselor than were Anglo-American girls.

Hanson found it helpful to include families when counseling adolescents.[55] Support from family members is solicited, building on the "instinct" of the adolescent to seek support and approval from the family. Ackerman has recommended that families generally be included in the counseling of sexually delinquent adolescents.[56] However, family therapists tend to recommend family treatment for ideological reasons rather than pragmatic ones. We might wonder how the pregnant adolescent will react to the inclusion of family members in what she originally considered her own counseling.

Baptiste advanced six reasons for family-focused counseling with adolescent pregnancies:

1. *The family's need to deal with its pervasive sense of failure precipitated by the pregnancy. . . .*

2. *Family members' need to clarify their different views about the pregnancy and the unborn baby. . . .*

3. *The need for the adolescent and her parents to resolve any conflicts existing prior to the pregnancy, and especially those resulting from the pregnancy situation. . . .*

4. *The importance of maintaining and/or improving communication in a crisis situation for the adolescent and her family. . . .*

5. *Parents' need to maintain their relationship while they "parent" their daughter through the crisis of pregnancy. . . .*

6. *Parents' and adolescents' need to resolve developmental independency-dependency issues.*[57]

He recommended a pragmatic approach to family counseling that embodied nine guidelines. Essentially, Baptiste urged counselors to be active and focused, avoiding consistent advocacy for any individual, and helping the family arrive at a solution that they could live with.

After a thorough review of the literature concerning the treatment of pregnant teens, Bolton recommended four goals for the counseling of pregnant adolescents and their families.[58] The first goal was to increase communication within the family. Action-oriented techniques such as role-playing were recommended as being compatible with families in the lower socioeconomic class who make up the majority of (but certainly not all) pregnant teens. The second goal was to establish or re-establish self-esteem within the adolescent and the members of the family. The trauma of an unplanned pregnancy was assumed to lower the self-esteem of virtually all family members, and communication techniques were recommended to help family members deal with their conflicts rather than bury them. The third goal was to educate the entire family about the pregnancy. The final goal was to educate the family about how they must pull together cooperatively as a team to cope with the crisis of pregnancy. Bolton recommended periodic crisis intervention for the emotional upheavals that inevitably occur throughout the pregnancy.

Possibilities

When a family comes to counseling, they will probably disagree with each other and with you over the best resolution of the pregnancy. The possibilities are limited to six: (1) girl and parents both want to bear the child to term; (2) girl wants to bear to term while parents are divided; (3) girl wants to bear to term while both parents recommend abortion; (4) girl and parents both want abortion; (5) girl wants abortion while parents are divided; (6) girl wants abortion and parents both want her to bear to term. The same divisions are possible regardless of the decision to be made—adoption, living at home, marriage of the adolescent, or other related decisions.

In the following sections, I will assume that the counselor cannot—and should not, even if it were possible—be value free. A counselor must inevitably believe something. If the counselor believes that whatever the counselees decide is fine, the counselor is still taking a value stance.

Counselors realize that counselees *will* make free choices. Some counselees will inevitably make unwise and even sinful choices. So do counselors. Proper ethical practice by the counselor is to make sure that the counselees understand his or her values so that statements will not be thought value free when they are value loaded. Counselees need to be able to understand the counselor's actions and recommendations within the context of the counselor's value system.

I believe that life begins at conception and that abortion can only be justified if the mother's life is endangered. In that instance, the choice is whether both lives will be lost or only one life. Although not everyone who reads this book will agree with my position, I will write this section according to my beliefs while respecting the perspectives of those who hold other positions.

Everyone agrees to bear to term. In only one of the six possible scenarios will all participants agree. In that instance— where everyone wants the girl to bear to term—the counselor will concentrate his or her efforts on (a) dealing with the emotional reactions of family members to the pregnancy, (b) attending to details of the pregnancy such as getting proper health care and nutrition for the mother, and (c) planning how each family member can support the mother throughout the pregnancy.

The counselor must be alert to unresolved blame and unforgiveness of family members. Within the church, there is a strong norm that families should pull together in times of stress. This will increase the likelihood that Christian families will actually pull together, but will also result in many of the families being unwilling to admit that they are angry, disappointed and disillusioned with the girl for her pregnancy. Broach the issue of support early in counseling as you deal with the emotional reactions to the crisis. It is important, though, that you accept the family members' statements at face value. Encourage them to support the adolescent. However, as counseling progresses, stay alert for signs that family members blame the adolescent for family troubles. As specific instances of blame show up, you can more easily deal with them than you can by discussing blame early in counseling when family members are denying negative feelings toward their daughter.

Girl and one parent want the child; other parent wants abortion. In the second instance, where the girl and one parent want the girl to bear to term but one parent recommends abortion, conflict is inevitable. The danger is that you will throw your weight behind the girl's and agreeable parent's side and choke off the arguments of the other spouse. My recommendation is to ask the girl to explain her thoughts first. If the parents talk first and disagree, the girl will feel caught in the middle and will be reluctant to share her thoughts freely. The second person to share should be the parent who agrees with the girl. After that parent makes a case for bearing the baby to term, you might summarize the reasons adduced by the girl and the supportive parent. Then ask the other parent for his or her view.

How you respond to the conflict will depend on your assessment of the conflict. Is it long-standing conflict? If so, stay alert for another issue about which the parents disagree. If you find such an issue, you might suggest a compromise in which you support the parent recommending the baby be carried to term on that issue but support the other parent on the new issue. Even if the conflict is specific to the pregnancy situation and the family rules are generally stable, you must be sure that everyone is given a fair chance to speak.

Generally, the spouse who recommends abortion is concerned with the disruption in the life of the girl that will be caused by bearing the child to term. You can often introduce other information. For example, you might show that the psychological effects of an abortion are also disruptive—as disruptive as having the baby.[59] You can mention the possibility of adoption, which will provide an excellent home for the baby while not tying the adolescent down as a single parent. Using the method of Ury and Fisher,[60] identify the interests of the spouse who wants the girl to have an abortion. Try to get the spouse to identify those interests and propose ways that the interests might be satisfied without abortion.

Girl doesn't want abortion; parents do. The third situation, in which the girl wants to bear the baby to term while both parents want abortion, is potentially explosive. Try to avoid teaming up with the girl in opposition to both parents. Generally, the parents simply will not return to counseling if they feel that you do not support them. Rather, allow the girl to express her opinion first, then allow the parents to express their opinions. Describe the situation as an impasse. Try to avoid allowing the parents to pressure the girl to give in to their demands.

I generally say something like, "It seems that you have reached a stalemate. You, Karen, want to keep the baby safe and not have it killed. And you, Mr. and Mrs. Smith, are concerned about the difficulties and pain that having a child might cause for Karen and even for the whole family. Karen, you have a legitimate interest in the baby that is within you, and I know it is painful for you to disagree with your parents. Mr. and Mrs. Smith, you are justifiably concerned about your daughter, just as she is concerned with her child. It seems that there might be ways that we could satisfy both of these parental instincts. Of course, I know it is hard for you, Mr. and Mrs. Smith, to have your daughter disagree with you. As a parent, I certainly don't like it when my children disagree with me. But in this instance it sounds as if Karen is responding to her parental feelings just like you both are. Are there some ways that both sets of instincts can be handled? If we could put aside our emotions for a few minutes, we might come up with a way in which no one loses rather than imposing a solution in which there will be long-lasting pain. What do you think?"

Girl and parents want abortion. In the fourth situation, the girl and both parents want abortion. This situation is unlikely to occur because there is little reason for this family to attend counseling. Generally, if all family members agree about the abortion, they will get it before coming to counseling. However, if they do come to counseling, you will probably wish to express your opinion about abortion before counseling has proceeded very far. "I think that you should all know that I believe you would be making a mistake if you proceed with the abortion. There are a number of reasons from scripture that suggest that life has begun from conception (such as Ps. 139:13–16; Isa. 49:1; Jer. 1:5; Gal. 1:15), and I think you should read those before you make your final decision about the abortion. Aside from that, however, there are some other reasons that abortion is not such an easy solution to pregnancy as it at first seems. For example, abortion might hurt Karen's ability to conceive children later. Abortion also has had a number of psychological difficulties associated with it, too, such as guilt, depression and in some cases even suicide that occurs on the anniversary of the date of the abortion. You must make this decision using your best judgment, but I urge you to put it off for a week and read some of the writings about the effects of abortion. A week probably won't make much difference and it will give you a chance to satisfy yourself that you are making the best decision, so you won't later feel that you have rushed into a mistake."

Girl and one parent want abortion; other parent doesn't. In the fifth situation, the girl wants an abortion and she is supported by one parent but not the other. You must again carefully consider the long-standing balance of power and stability within the family. As with any division in power, look for another issue about which the parents disagree so that you can use it to suggest compromise. Allow the girl to give her reasons for abortion first so that she will not be caught in the middle any more than she already is. Then ask the parent who disagrees with the girl to express himself or herself. Finally, ask the other parent to give his or her reasons for supporting the girl. By dividing the two arguments for abortion, you weaken them and call attention to the conflict within the family rather than to the united front between the girl and one parent. After all participants have expressed their opinions, summarize by describing the obvious conflict. Again, appeal to the interests behind each position and try to seek ways that can meet both sets of interests.

Girl wants abortion; parents don't. In the sixth situation, where the girl wants an abortion but the parents want her to bear the child to term, your main concern is that the adolescent will feel that you are not supporting her and will therefore be reluctant to attend future counseling. You must help her understand that you understand her perspective and respect it. Call her attention to the long-term consequences of abortion and to the effects of the abortion on her family of origin, both of which early and middle adolescents are not likely to consider. Ask her to speculate about the alternatives to abortion and to imagine what it would be like in each instance. Help her examine positive as well as negative aspects of each alternative. Be sure to present the negative consequences likely from abortion as well as the ending of the pregnancy.

Pro-Life Arguments

During your discussions with the family, disagreements will result in many reasons given for abortion. Arguments against abortion have been detailed in many publications.[61] Some of the common proabortion arguments are succinctly mentioned below along with brief refutations.

1. *The fetus is not yet human.* R(refutation): What is it then? Before pregnancy is discovered, the unborn baby has a heartbeat and brainwaves.

2. *The fetus is potentially human but has no consciousness.* R: A sleeping adult also has no consciousness, nor does a person in a coma. Consciousness is not the *sine qua non* for life.

3. *The baby's quality of life will be low if it is born poor.* R: The sanctity of life is more important than the quality of life. Should all people who don't have a quality of life that *you* consider "good" be put to death?

4. *The fetus is part of the girl's body and she can do with it what she pleases.* R: The baby is merely being carried by the girl; it is genetically different from the girl.

5. *The baby cannot live apart from the girl.* R: If I am in jail, I cannot live apart from the jailer. Does this power over me give the jailer the moral right to take my life? Further, medical advances have progressed until babies born early in the middle trimester have lived.

6. *I don't want a baby.* R: Why not give it up for adoption? There are many thousands of couples who would be glad to love the child and give it an excellent home. There is no such thing as an unwanted child in many nations of the world today.

Remember that the counseling room is not a court of law or a public debate. Your motivation for giving reasons not to get an abortion is *not* to win an argument or to prove you are right. You can be thoroughly right and have the clients never return to counseling. The reason *is* to provide accurate information that family members can use to decide on a course of action that they can live with. It is not your responsibility to persuade the family to do things your way. It is your responsibility to help them consider options while being true to your own beliefs. Argue, when necessary, but with sensitivity and gentleness.

Crisis Counseling with Families of Adolescents

Leveton has recommended one way to handle counseling with families of adolescents in crisis.[62] She describes three stages of counseling. Usually the family will feel and demonstrate resistance to counseling because they feel forced to attend counseling by the crisis. The resistance might be shown as a direct challenge to the counselor. Or the resistance might be more subtle, such as engaging in almost endless talk about the problem but being reluctant to discuss what can be done about the problem. Other families simply refuse to discuss the problem, become lost in details, or act confused about the causes and solutions for the problem. Usually the counselor who is unprepared for the family's resistance will feel upset and disappointed. Forgetting the family's perception that a counselor is basically an outsider, the counselor might become angry at the family members for their resistance.

Rather, in the initial stage of counseling, the counselor must understand the resistance of the family as an expression of pain and fear. Other emotions such as guilt and shame also threaten to overwhelm family members. Secondly, the counselor must understand that the family needs help. The discovery of the pregnancy shocks and unbalances the family and disrupts its usual functioning.

Generally, the counselor must be warm, friendly, and accepting. Speak to every member of the family in the early stage of counseling so that no one feels left out. Lead the family away from blaming and shaming, and stress the importance of expressing feelings and checking out family members' assumptions.

Leveton recommends that the counselor try to understand

how family members usually relate to each other. She decries the belief that crisis intervention is *merely* to help the family solve their problems, saying that without some understanding about the dynamics of the family, many solutions will be undermined by the family.

Armed with a rudimentary understanding of the family, the counselor can then determine which part of the crisis can be resolved in the few sessions of crisis counseling that are available. The counselor must explicitly establish goals for crisis sessions or the family will become disappointed in the counseling. The counselor then formulates short-term plans to handle the parts of the crisis that will be addressed. Usually, three or four sessions are sufficient to address the main issues in the crisis.

Leveton recommends that the counselor not try to adopt a style that he or she thinks might be effective with the family. Rather, she assumes that the counselor's best resource is himself or herself and his or her natural style. Counseling is generally task-oriented, with an explicit contract.

Involving the Baby's Father

The baby's father will become involved in several counseling situations. Usually he will not be involved formally with the decision about the resolution of the pregnancy unless marriage is being considered, though the adolescent usually strongly considers his opinion. When marriage is being considered, sessions that involve the pregnant adolescent, the father of the child, and both families of the girl and the boy may be helpful.

A second situation that commonly involves the father of the child is after marriage. The couple, who usually struggle with their relationship, might request counseling either before or after the birth of the child, especially if the counselor has been helpful in the decision to bear the child to term.

A third situation that often involves the father of the baby is when the adolescent girl and the father decide not to marry and then she decides to place the child for adoption. They may differ in their opinions about whether to place the child for adoption. Disagreements can also occur over the name of the child (the child cannot be given the last name of the father without his signature) and over whether to place the child through a private or public adoption agency.

Generally, if counseling is sought because the adolescent and the baby's father disagree over pregnancy resolution, the name of the child, or adoption agreements, you will support the mother and help the girl and boy express their feelings and arrive at some understanding about how things will be. Compromise might not be necessary or even desirable in many cases.

If the couple seek marriage counseling, that counseling will differ little from your usual marriage counseling. I have written about how to counsel married Christians in a separate work.[63] The only difference is that the counselor must remain especially attentive to external pressures and demands that weigh on the adolescent couple. Often their relationship is under considerable strain because they lack basic interpersonal skills, maturity, or economic opportunity. Many times the work of the counselor with the adolescent couple involves practical assistance such as phoning welfare, helping the couple live on their budget—or even creating a budget—helping the adolescents learn interviewing and job-seeking skills, and helping them resolve conflicts by simply seeing the other person's perspective.

PREVENTION OF TEEN PREGNANCY

Short of the second coming of Christ, teen pregnancy probably cannot be prevented. It will occur. The concerned Christian—whether pastor, professional counselor, parent, elder, or lay person within the congregation—can contribute to decreasing its incidence.

Adolescents must learn about sex. However, learning through the schools, which try to present sex education within the context of individual choice, does not decrease teenage pregnancy. A good case can be made that it *increases* teen pregnancy.[64] Rather, to decrease teen pregnancy, sex education must occur within a clearly *moral* context.[65] Decisions about premarital sexual intercourse and about abortion are *moral* decisions, not lifestyle decisions. At present, most learning about the mechanics of sex takes place through peers and media (movies and magazines). Parents and churches must become more involved in the sex education of young people.

Schools, too, can be involved in sex education. But not as they are currently involved. Rather than being dispensers of sexual information and secular values, or even worse, sites of comprehensive health care clinics in which families give blanket permission for their child to receive any kind of health care (including contraceptive and abortion information), schools can be training grounds *for parents of adolescents*. Programs might be offered that include information about sexuality to parents along with coaching about how to communicate that information effectively to their children. Extension services, much like the home economics extension services which brought nutritional information to lower socioeconomic families, could be established to go into communities and show families how to educate their own children about sexuality. In that way, parents could transmit accurate information to their children within the context of the family's values.

From the research on transmission of religious values to adolescents, we know that parents can more effectively transmit their values to their children if the home is characterized by warmth, acceptance, low levels of parent-child and marital conflict, and firm but loving control of children. Churches and individuals can thus help prevent teenage pregnancy by building positive environments within the homes of adolescents.

Adolescents can be armed, too, with skills for self-control. These involve learning to say no to peers and dates who promote nonmarital sexual expression. Adolescents, too, can develop strategies to focus their attention on the long-term benefits of chastity and long-term consequences of premarital sex. Many adolescents say they engaged in premarital sex because they found no good reasons for saying no. Adolescents can be helped to see that there *are* good reasons for deferring sex until marriage.

Finally, adolescents can be shown how to claim the promise of God that "No temptation has overtaken you that is not common to man. God is faithful, and he will not let you be tempted beyond your strength, but with the temptation will also provide the way of escape, that you may be able to endure it"

(1 Cor. 10:13). The time to claim that promise is not in the back seat of a car with the clothes half removed. Rather, it is before agreeing to go to the parking place where a difficult decision might arise.

TEENAGE MOTHERS

Early investigations of mothering during adolescence claimed that teen mothers had infants who were more at risk than infants of mothers in their twenties. Furthermore, maternal mortality was thought to be greater for teen mothers than for nonteen mothers. Later reviews[66] and studies have questioned the claim that infant and maternal mortality risk was directly proportional to age of the mother. Rather, fetal mortality of women thirty-five and older was found to be much higher than for women under twenty. Maternal mortality risk was over ten times as high for women over thirty-five than for adolescents.

This does not mean that teen parents are not at risk for difficulties. They clearly are. However, the risks are associated more with the socioeconomic status and physical size of the adolescent which is a covariant with the age of adolescents rather than being directly attributable to age itself. The same has been found with parenting skills. Generally, teen mothers have shown difficulties is using mature skills at mothering. However, research has shown that this is probably more related to the socioeconomic status of the mothers than to their age.

Nonetheless, motherhood is not easy.[67] Nor is fatherhood.[68] Yet, helping teenage mothers become mature parents is an important responsibility of the family of the adolescent and of the church. Rather than spend time coaching the teen mother about proper mothering, the counselor might concentrate on establishing a support network for the girl within the congregation. Mothers with experience—those with wise eyes, red hands, and happy infants of their own—can provide excellent models for young mothers. Because the power dynamics of a family are generally not present in friendships, many teen mothers are better able to learn from friends than from their own mothers.

The teen mother will be especially aided by practical books

and tapes that teach through concrete example. A few of the better books are listed in Appendix 1.

COUNSELING FOR ADOPTION

When an adolescent has carried an infant for nine months and gone through labor to deliver the child, there is a strong bond between mother and child.[69] She is reluctant to break that bond, especially since the soaring divorce rate has made single motherhood so commonplace without accompanying social stigma.[70] Thus, over 95 percent of pregnant adolescents who bear their children to term decide to rear the child themselves.

Many adolescents decide to raise their own children for reasons they will regret in later years. Sometimes the teen mother thinks of the baby as someone who will love her. Seeking love and approval, the teen hopes that the child will provide that. It is not long before the adolescent learns the other side of love. The child demands sacrifice from the parent. The pleasures of changing diapers and getting up in the middle of the night somehow may not quite seem to make up for the costs. The adolescent can become disillusioned and reject the child.

Sometimes grandparents pressure the adolescent to raise the child because they cannot stand to "lose my grandchild." The adolescent has disappointed her parents once by becoming pregnant and is reluctant to disappoint them again by placing the child for adoption. Often the grandparents who pressure the adolescent to raise the child will become overinvolved in the parenting of the child. The adolescent initially enjoys the help she obtains with the mundane duties of motherhood. Later, resentments build, for the grandparents begin to feel a sense of ownership because of sacrifices they have made for the child. Vicious power struggles can arise.

Due to the adolescent mother's egocentric thinking ("things happen for *my* benefit and pleasure"), she might initially regard the infant as a pretty plaything. Sometimes, as the demands for child care mount, the adolescent becomes neglectful of the child. Many of the same factors which predict teenage pregnancy also predict child abuse and neglect. Bolton[71] has suggested that these factors *cause* child abuse in teen mothers, although his conclusions are not shared by most researchers.[72]

Adolescent mothers who elect to raise their child without being prepared for some of the costs that they will encounter are likely to be disappointed and disillusioned. Sometimes the counselor can steer them toward placing the child for adoption.

When the adolescent decides to give the child up for adoption, the adolescent will experience the grief of loss. The maternal-child bond is ruptured and feelings of loss, depression, and grief are common. The mother can generally console herself, though, by thinking that even if she feels a sense of sadness, the child will be happy in his or her new home. Couples are well screened so that there is a great likelihood that they will be excellent parents. The mother is allowed to specify the type of family that she would like to be considered as parents. For example, a Christian girl might request that the child be given to Christian parents and that request is generally honored. If the adolescent gives the baby to a private adoption service, arrangements can even be made for the mother to meet the parents before the adoption is formally completed. There is some suggestion that this helps the adoptive mother adjust to the loss of her baby more easily than if the adoptive parents are never met.

As a counselor, you might have to help the girl move through the stages of grief—from denial and numbed shock, to the phase in which she talks about the loss repetitively and compulsively and has doubts and misgivings about her action, until the final stage of acceptance. You might also have to deal with the loss by the family members of the adolescent. Books recommended for adjusting to adoption and for making a decision to place the child for adoption are given in Appendix 1.

CONCLUSION

Teenage pregnancy involves three generations of family members in decisions that are value laden and emotional. There are no easy answers to treating or reducing teenage pregnancy. The counselor must understand the dynamics of family operation under stress, the cognitive and moral development of the adolescent, the styles of decision making that are likely to be encountered in crisis situations, and specific information about pregnancy, childbirth, and motherhood.

Faced with great demands for skill and knowledge, the counselor who deals with the pregnant adolescent and her family usually feels incompetent and inadequate. Even preparing for counseling adolescents and honing one's skills leaves the counselor bewildered and overwhelmed at times. Caught between conflicting parties making necessary moral decisions, the counselor often feels defensive and disappointed when families make decisions with which the counselor disagrees.

The inadequacy we all feel in these situations can threaten to overwhelm us. In fact, once I simply had to stop a counseling session with a young family and put my head down in prayer. Although at the time I felt that the problems of the family had defeated me, I now see that situation as the turning point in my counseling. I came to the end of myself and had to rely totally on the Lord. Once I stopped pushing my agenda, Jesus was able to get into the family and work out the solution. Adolescent pregnancy is truly a problem requiring God's solution.

CHAPTER FIVE

COHABITING . . . AND PREGNANT

NONMARITAL HETEROSEXUAL COHABITATION IS USUALLY DEFINED as living together and engaging in regular sexual intercourse while unmarried. These living arrangements are increasingly practiced by more couples.[1] Macklin, almost ten years ago, estimated that approximately one-quarter of all college students cohabited at some time during their college career.[2] Watson estimated that over half of the people who now marry have previously cohabited with someone.[3] Nor is this merely true of "the world." Young couples in the church sometimes elect to cohabit, though strong prohibitions against cohabitation in most churches make it difficult to guess how often this occurs.

It has always been difficult to estimate the incidence of co-habitation. Because many people disapprove of cohabitation, some cohabiting couples lie about their living status, which reduces the number of cohabiting couples detected by census. On the other hand, census data do not include "unmarried cohabitation" as a distinct category. If an elderly woman rents rooms to college boys, the census will report unmarried males and females living in the same house, which increases apparent incidences of cohabitation. Despite inaccuracies in census data, it appears clear that nonmarital cohabitation is rising yearly.[4]

WHY DISCUSS COHABITATION?

Some social scientists advocate cohabitation as a legitimate lifestyle.[5] Often their reasoning boils down to the argument that cohabitation is widespread so we should accept it. This is an example of *is*-to-*ought* reasoning—i.e., what *is* should be. Until recently, such reasoning has been morally repugnant to most people. For instance, Marquis de Sade used is-to-ought reasoning. He said that men are stronger than women, thus men ought to be able to use women as they wish. Recently, though, anthropologists, sociologists, and psychologists have generally preached moral relativism, which is undergirded with the presupposition that because a variety of behavior patterns exist, we should accept each of them. Berger and Berger, in a masterful book defending the family as an institution, have traced the impact of culturally relativistic thinking on the way that the definition of the family has changed.[6]

In 1980, plans to celebrate the "Year of the Family" led to a position paper by Hutchinson.[7] He argued that the concept of the nuclear family as the normative American family while all other family constellations are called broken families is outmoded. He suggested instead that the idea of "the family" be replaced with the concept of "families," which would include single-parent families, reconstituted families, cohabiting families, and even homosexual families. Berger and Berger describe the conflict that erupted over that change of definition, culminating with Senator Paul Laxalt's Family Protection Act. The Bergers argued that new forms of the family should not be accepted as normative simply because they existed. Rather, the normative standard of the nuclear family should be retained as the defining element of society.

My position concerning cohabitation (or adolescent pregnancy, for that matter) is that I do not approve of it. I recognize it as a problem of social and individual morality and as a situation leading to pain which as a Christian I am called upon to fight. Like unmarried adolescent pregnancy, the unmarried pregnancy of cohabiting couples stems from sinful sexual intercourse. I can legitimately hate that sin, yet accept the sinners—even "while we (they) are yet sinners" (Rom. 5:8). As a Christian, I will, of course, gently and compassionately call them to repentance for their own benefit if I can do so lovingly in a way that they can hear.

CAUSES OF COHABITATION

As with any phenomenon, causes can be described on many different levels. Societal causes of cohabitation include the rise in divorce rate, leaving many divorced people who have been hurt by their spouses and who try to avoid a repetition of that hurt by living together rather than marrying again. Even among the elderly, the rate of cohabitation has increased. Often elderly couples can live together and collect more individual government benefits than they could if they were married. At the same time the cost of maintaining one household is less than the cost of maintaining two. College-age couples often use a similar economic argument to justify their cohabitation. Another societal cause for the rise in cohabitation is its increasing acceptability to a variety of people, reflecting the erosion of Judeo-Christian moral standards.

On the psychological level more people are engaging in cohabitation because of the increasing emphasis on individuality and pleasure-seeking without commitment. Kohlberg described six stages of moral development.[8] Young adults and late adolescents, who usually are in the first three stages of moral development, are especially attracted to cohabitation. In Kohlberg's first stage, the fear of punishment controls moral action. Adolescents who operate using predominately stage 1 moral reasoning use the feeling of freedom that they gain once they move away from their parents' residence to legitimate their decision to cohabit. Their parents cannot discover their living arrangements, so they feel free from punishment.

The second stage of moral development is based on hedonism. The late adolescent or early adult who operates primarily from stage 2 moral reasoning is likely to justify cohabitation because it "feels right." The person might say, "We are in love. It feels so right to be together. But neither of us feels that we are mature enough for a lifetime commitment of marriage, so we are living together." Those who operate mostly according to stage 3 moral reasoning will justify their actions according to what they perceive authorities say is right. Numerous different authorities might be invoked in their justification. Most late adolescents who cohabit believe that their parents would support their cohabitation if asked. They frequently deceive themselves into believing that their parents believe as they do.[9] Other late adolescents cite their professors, certain authors, or the vast majority of their peers as the "authority" who justifies their actions.

Besides societal and psychological causes of cohabitation, the increasing incidence of AIDS and of sexually transmitted diseases (STD) such as herpes, gonorrhea, syphilis, and other forms of venereal diseases has contributed to increasing cohabitation. With the promiscuous sexual behavior of the 1970s, STD has become an epidemic. Nurtured on sexual permissiveness but leary of STD, late adolescents and early adults of the 1980s are prone to opt for monogamy in premarital sexual relationships rather than for premarital chastity.

Finally, the decision to cohabit depends greatly on how people define cohabitation—as a life-style issue or as a moral issue. Worthington and Danser examined the effects of religious beliefs and of perceived parental values on statements of willingness to cohabit in late adolescents.[10] As with other studies, they found a moderate correlation between religious beliefs and unwillingness to cohabit and between perceived parental attitudes opposing cohabitation and the unwillingness to cohabit. However, they found that a much stronger relationship existed between how adolescents defined cohabitation—as a life-style issue or as a moral issue—and the willingness to

cohabit. Adolescents who held strong religious beliefs and perceived their parents to oppose cohabitation defined the cohabitation decision as a moral one; once that decision was made,
adolescents usually said they were unwilling to cohabit. Adolescents who were not religious and perceived their parents as
not opposing cohabitation usually defined cohabitation as a
life-style issue and were willing to cohabit. This suggests that
an insidious effect of defining cohabitation is that it becomes
simply an alternative lifestyle. Cultural acceptance of that
definition in many schools and in some governmental actions
has led to increasing acceptance that cohabitation is something
one *should* be willing to consider.

EFFECTS OF COHABITATION ON MARRIAGE STABILITY

People who cohabit often argue that cohabitation is good
preparation for marriage. Some view cohabitation as a trial
marriage to see whether they are compatible with their partners. Others view cohabitation as a way of building relationship skills which presumably generalize to marriage.

Research studies show the opposite, that cohabitation has a
negative effect on marriage. Several studies have compared
couples who cohabited and then were married with couples
who married without prior cohabitation. The results are summarized in Table 3. All these studies show that the divorce
and marital dissatisfaction rate in married couples who have
and who have not cohabited prior to marriage either are equal
or that cohabiting couples have higher divorce rates and more
marital dissatisfaction than noncohabiting couples.

This is amazing. Couples who lived together for a while and
then decided *not* to marry because they were in some way
"incompatible" were not even considered in the group of cohabiting couples. Thus, couples with presumably less sexual experience and less daily knowledge about their spouse at the
time of marriage have fewer divorces than couples who cohabited and then married.

Two speculations have been advanced to explain these findings. Newcomb suggested that couples who cohabit are less
inhibited by social norms than the noncohabitors, as evidenced
by their willingness to go against the social norm prohibiting

114

A Comparison of Findings in Research Comparing Couples Who Did (C) and Did Not Cohabit (NC) Prior to Marriage[11]

Author(s)	Date	Participants	Findings
Bentler & Newcomb	1978	77 couples (4 years after marriage)	Divorce rate after 4 years (C = NC)
Jacques & Chason	1979	University students C = 54; NC = 30	Sexual satisfaction (C = NC) Relationship stability (C = NC) Physical intimacy (C = NC) Openness of communication (C = NC)
Bentler & Newcomb	1980a	68 couples married 4 years from Los Angeles	Marital satisfaction (C = NC)
Newcomb & Bentler	1980b	159 couples from Los Angeles	Related to marital longevity: Males: attractiveness (-), religious commitment,(+) masculinity (+) Females: religious background (+), history of divorce (-), interest in art (-), attractiveness (-), introversion (+), intelligence (-), law abidance (+), clothes consciousness (+), religious commitment (+), femininity (+), conservatism (+), leadership (-)
Watson	1983	161 couples, mostly noncollege	Dyadic adjustment (NC > C); this was especially true for females but not for males
DeMaris	1984	309 recently married couples; 187 first marriage, 122 second marriage	Husbands, marital satisfaction for first marriages but not remarriages (NC > C)
DeMaris & Leslie	1984	General sample in Gainesville, Florida, recently married couples (N = 309)	Wives, marital satisfaction for first marriages but not remarriages (NC > C) Quality of communication, wives (NC > C) Quality of communication, husbands (C = NC) Marital satisfaction, wives (NC > C) Marital satisfaction, husbands (even when controlling for church attendance, sex role traditionalism, others, (NC > C)

Table 3

115

cohabitation.[12] Thus, he reasons, cohabiting couples might be expected to be less inhibited by norms against divorce. This reasoning is questionable on a number of accounts. First, the divorce rate is well over 50 percent[13] and, if Watson's estimate is accurate, over half of the people cohabit before marriage.[14] Then the assumption that societal norms prohibit cohabitation and divorce is incorrect. In fact, there are two societal norms. One set discourages cohabitation and divorce and the other set permits them. The societal norm, thus, depends on the subgroup of society with which a person identifies. On college campuses, one might argue that the predominant social norms encourage cohabitation and that the college student who decides not to cohabit is the one standing against social norms. Second, our research[15] showed that late adolescents chose whether to cohabit or not depending on the values they perceived to be held by their parents. Thus, instead of standing against social norms, late adolescents merely showed that two sets of parental norms were being perceived—one set accepting cohabitation and another set not accepting cohabitation.

A second speculation about why cohabitation tends to lead to higher divorce rates than with couples who have not cohabited was advanced by Kotkin,[16] who suggested that cohabiting couples expect to cohabit only as long as they are sure they love each other. Despite the vows taken when these couples later marry, Kotkin thinks that the expectation continues after marriage, "As long as we both shall love." This thinking makes divorce likely.

A third speculation is that cohabiting and noncohabiting couples differ in religious beliefs.[17] Religious couples tend to divorce less often than nonreligious couples. Thus, if religious couples were removed from both groups, then divorce rates might be equal for couples who had and who had not cohabited.

TRANSITION FROM COHABITATION TO MARRIAGE

Couples who are cohabiting or who are willing to cohabit usually view cohabitation as similar to marriage. They expect little if any difference in the relationship after they marry. That usually leads to a rude surprise.

Charles and Cathy were cohabiting and intending to marry.

One week before the marriage, if you were to ask Charles and Cathy why they were together, they would reply almost in unison, "because we love each other."

One week after the marriage, if you were to pose the same question to them, "Why are you together?" they would answer, "because we are married."

Nothing changed except the ceremony, yet the way Charles and Cathy thought about their relationship was altered. This would importantly influence the couple's ability to resolve conflicts.

In addition, at marriage Charles and Cathy experience changes in their economic status. They can now file their income tax return as a married couple, which will change the amount of income tax they pay and the amount of income tax withheld from each paycheck. They also will probably experience a lessening of disapproval from the authority figures in their lives. Their parents will be more accepting of their relationship, and their relationship more acceptable in God's eyes, too, which will lessen their feelings of guilt.

EFFECT OF PREGNANCY DURING COHABITATION

Despite their use of birth control, Cathy became pregnant before marriage. With the pregnancy came social disapproval. There was open criticism by family, friends, co-workers, and employers. The strong social pressure to legitimate the birth of their child forced them to consider the future of the relationship.

Cathy first decided she would get an abortion. She secretly went to Planned Parenthood for the "procedure." When she arrived, however, her conscience began to bother her and she cancelled the appointment. After talking with Charles, Cathy agreed to see their pastor and seek his counsel about the abortion. Although they attended a rather liberal church, Charles and Cathy were surprised that their pastor recommended not having an abortion. He took a much more conservative stand than they expected, referring to the fetus as the "life growing within Cathy's womb." At the end of the hour and one-half session with the pastor, Cathy and Charles decided to bear the child to term. Although they had been surprised that the pastor had not recommended the abortion when they described the difficulties that their child would create for them, they were also relieved that they did not have to obtain the abortion. It was one thing to talk about abortion in abstract discussions while in college, but it was much more difficult to actually have it.

When the news came out in the congregation, the members were surprisingly (to Charles and Cathy) accepting and supportive. Some disapproved and clearly showed it. One older woman pointed her finger at them during Bible study and described the sinfulness and shame they should be feeling. After her harangue, she sat down, shut her eyes, and removed her hearing aid. Nonetheless, most people in the congregation made a "fuss" over the new mother—even giving her a shower.

Once they had decided to bear the child to term, four choices were open to them. They might continue to cohabit and simply put up with increased disapproval from their friends and church family. Or they might decide that the relationship had no future and that Cathy should raise the child as a single parent. They knew that a single mother would experience less disapproval than a cohabiting couple with a child. The third option was to give the child up for adoption. The fourth option was to marry and raise the child. Together they decided to place the child for adoption.

CHRISTMAS GIFT

A nurse on the labor and delivery floor described to me what happened to Charles and Cathy.

Three days before Christmas, they checked into the hospital. Cathy was in labor. Even though they were not married, they delivered in the "birthing room" and gave birth to a healthy baby girl. They had attended Lamaze classes together, supporting each other—so young, so far away from both sets of parents.

On the first day after delivery, Cathy asked me to bring her girl to her. "Are you sure you want to hold her, honey?" I asked, knowing that she had already decided to place the child for adoption. She was placing the child at the Catholic Adoption House. Once she left the hospital, Cathy would have a month to reclaim her child before it was adoptable.

"Sure, bring the little brat to me. She means nothing to me. I don't want her. I just want to hold and feed her."

She held the baby at arm's length and frowned at it. "You're ugly," she said. "I don't love you. I hate you. Here, take this bottle, you homely creature. You'll never amount to anything."

At every feeding, she repeated the ritual. All the other nurses on the floor watched with the same morbid fascination that I did. It was so obvious that she loved the child. Yet she was determined to continue with her own life, unencumbered by a child. She would tell the child repeatedly that she was a millstone, a weight that dragged her down, a burden.

At four o'clock every afternoon after work, Charles would visit. He would sit on the side of the bed and look fondly at Cathy. Bits of conversation would float toward me when I worked in their room. "Just stand in the way of our careers," Cathy would say. "Are you sure you want to go through with this?" Charles would ask time and time again. "Are you positive?"

After visiting hours were ended, I saw Charles standing outside the nursery, his arm pressed against the glass and his head leaning against his arm. Staring at the baby.

Just before leaving at 11 that night, I looked in on Cathy. She was softly crying. "What's wrong?"

"Nothing. I'm fine."

"Can I get you anything?"

"No."

The nurses on the night shift said that Cathy got little sleep that night. Yet the next day, when Charles came by after work, the scene of the previous day was repeated. He sat on the bed asking whether she was really sure she was doing what she wanted to do. Coldly, she assured him that she didn't want the baby, never had, and never would. In my opinion, she was protecting Charles, and he was protecting her. The entire staff of nurses was upset. Two sensitive people, in love with each other, were giving each other the gift of the Magi, sacrificing their child.

The last I saw of Charles on Christmas Eve night he was looking at the child through the nursery window. Cathy was crying as I left work. On Christmas, the nurses on the morning shift told me that Cathy had coldly left the hospital, leaving her baby for the Catholic Adoption Home. As she walked away arm in arm with Charles, she never looked back. Together they went off to their careers.

Two weeks later, Sue, the head nurse at the nurse's station answered the phone. Solemnly she placed the receiver in its cradle and turned to face us. She cleared her throat. "That was the Catholic Adoption Home. Cathy and Charles took home their little girl."

Every nurse at the station cheered.

Charles and Cathy had given belated Christmas gifts all around.

THE DECISION TO MARRY

Once Cathy and Charles decided to marry, there were still many issues to work out between them. They had to change their attitudes toward each other to emphasize their commitment. The decision to marry also affected Charles and Cathy's attributions about why they were living together. Now the answers are many: "Because we had to get married." "Because we are married." "Because of the child—to give her legitimacy and a good environment to grow up in." "Because we love each other." "Because we were pressured."

Given the many ways that the couple can explain their life together, Charles and Cathy might have difficulties resolving any troubles they are likely to have.

COUNSELING THE PREGNANT COHABITING COUPLE

During the time from which the pregnancy is discovered by a cohabiting couple until after the marriage and childbirth, the couple might request counseling. There are numerous decision points, as in adolescent pregnancy; however, with the cohabiting couple, the couple is usually older and more independent of their parents than are adolescents. Much of your counseling will likely be with the couple and will not involve the families of origin. Generally, the higher maturity of the couple will mean that they will come to counseling for specific help rather than attend counseling throughout the entire pregnancy. Thus, rather than describe counseling throughout the pregnancy, I will describe several discrete interventions that the counselor might make.

Dealing with Blame for the Pregnancy

When pregnancy is a surprise during cohabitation, as it was with Charles and Cathy, generally the couple seeks counseling believing that someone is to blame for the pregnancy. Charles and Cathy used the diaphragm as their method of birth control. On the day that she got pregnant, Charles came home from work and caught Cathy in the bathtub. The bantering soon turned to sex play. Charles suggested that they stop to get the diaphragm, which was upstairs. Cathy playfully said, "Don't stop," and intercourse followed. Later, Cathy said that she had assumed that Charles would withdraw before ejaculation. He said that he assumed Cathy knew that the time of the month was safe. Although the accusations were not bitter, both were clearly pointing the finger at the other.

In fact, Charles and Cathy were pointing the finger at about everyone they knew. They blamed their church friends for being so narrow-minded about abortion. They blamed God for allowing them to get pregnant. They blamed their pastor for the counsel he gave about having the child. They blamed their parents for the way they were raised. Although they did not admit it, they blamed themselves for giving in to a few moments of fun and pleasure instead of taking the precaution of birth control that they knew they needed to take.

The counselor's role was to divert their attention from blame to handling the problems they will face at the following stages. When couples blame someone for their problems, they assume that if they could determine the main cause for the problem, the problems will automatically disappear. This is clearly not the case. Blaming is employed to avoid facing decision making. If the couple cannot agree on who is *really* to blame, they can allow decisions to be made by default and then, in retrospect, blame the other person for failing to make the decision. A counselor needs to focus the couple's attention away from blame and draw it continually to the impending decisions. For example, the pastor who counseled Charles and Cathy to bear the child to term rather than abort diverted Charles and Cathy from blaming and got them working as a team throughout the remainder of the pregnancy. Here is part of their conversation.

Cathy (to Charles): Listen, *you* should have taken the responsibility for making sure that we didn't get pregnant. You could have stopped it. You knew we didn't have that diaphragm in.

Charles: Come on. You didn't say one word about there being any danger that we would get pregnant. Sometimes I think you wanted to get pregnant. You've always wanted to get married, and I think you just saw your chance.

Pastor Bob: Just a minute. I'm getting the picture in listening to you over the last few minutes that you each think the other stayed at home all day thinking up ways that you could get pregnant. Maybe you even stayed up all night the previous night planning your strategies, too. But that is a very different idea than I had when you started talking about the pregnancy. When you first began, it sounded like you had decided that you had a problem that the two of you had to solve together. Now, I understand that you each feel upset about the pregnancy—like it is unfair and like you wish it hadn't happened. I understand the anger and frustration of being stuck with it and not feeling like there is anything you can do that will provide a way out of the difficulty. That's confusing. There are a lot of thoughts and feelings trapped in each of you. Thoughts and feelings that are at odds with each other. But if you continue to blame the other person, I would predict that you won't get very far in deciding what you want to do next about this life growing within you.

Cathy: I know you're right, Pastor Bob. I know Charles didn't *mean* to have us get pregnant. I'm just sick about it.

Charles: It is a problem. I'm upset and confused, and I don't know what we ought to do. Cathy tried to get an abortion, but we thought we ought to talk about it a little more. That's why we are here today.

Pastor Bob, having been through many crises in his thirty-four years of ministry, wisely got Charles and Cathy away from blame and defined the task of counseling as problem solving. But he also acknowledged the emotional difficulty for both Cathy and Charles, showing that he understood what they were going through in their emotional lives. After they talked about their feelings, they were better able to approach their difficulty as a problem to solve.

Confronting the Cohabitation as Sin

John White described the need to confront a couple engaged in habitual sexual sin.[18] As a physician and psychiatrist, he used a medical analogy. He said that if a patient has cancer, the patient needs to be told. The loving and compassionate act of the physician is not to pretend that the patient has nothing wrong but to tell the patient about the cancer and its danger to life. The person can then make a decision about whether or not to have surgery to remove the cancer. The surgery is liable to be painful and require months or even years of healing and rehabilitation. However, the cancer left untreated will ultimately prove fatal.

Of course, the *way* in which a physician tells the painful news to the patient is crucial. In the old joke, a Marine drill sergeant found out about the death of the mother of Smith, a new recruit. The Marine pondered over graceful ways of breaking the sad news. Finally, he assembled the troops and hastily said, "All soldiers with living mothers take one step forward. Not so fast, Smith!" Sensitive.

Although the joke is somewhat perverse, I have seen well-meaning counselors confront people about sin with similar insensitivity. Sometimes we evangelical Christians can be the most insensitive precisely *because* we have the standard of God's Word that tells us that our counselee is sinning.

But a physician who knows that the patient absolutely has cancer must tell the patient in a way that the patient can understand. Also, we must tell the cohabiting couple that their sex outside of marriage is against the character of God and do so in a way that the couple can understand. Our task is to speak the truth in love (Eph. 4:15). It is the task of the Holy Spirit to convince the couple to change.

There is no single way to tell a couple that their cohabitation is sin. With some couples, it is necessary to be direct and blunt. With other couples, you must affirm their positive motives but show them that cohabitation is still not in line with God's Word.

The couple might not be willing to renounce their cohabitation as sin or they might acknowledge it as sin but decide to continue. That would force the counselor to make a hard decision. Some counselors refuse to counsel a couple who continue to engage in willful sin. They see an ongoing counseling relationship with the couple as encouraging (or at best tacitly approving of) the couple in sin (Rom. 1:32). They want to initiate church discipline procedures against the couple (Matt. 18:15–17; 1 Cor. 5:2b–5). Other counselors might continue to work with the couple. They argue that the counselor can make it plain that he or she does not approve of cohabitation, thus allowing the Holy Spirit to work. The counselor is obviously not encouraging or tacitly approving of the sin. Counselors might also argue that although the couple is sinning through cohabitation, they are not sinning against the counselor (Matt. 18:15a—"If your brother *sins against you* . . .") and are therefore not candidates for church discipline. The counterargument is that the man in Corinth who was sinning by living with his father's wife (1 Cor. 5:2–5; 2 Cor. 2:5–11) was not sinning against Paul, but Paul nonetheless recommended that the man be disciplined. The argument will then turn on the nature of public, disgraceful sin. Whether the couple's conduct is a public scandal that reflects poorly on the church will depend on the situation and on the interpretations of the Christian community.

How the counselor will behave if the couple rejects his or her advice is not a simple matter for me to decide—though some feel it is simple for them. It is a matter of scriptural interpretation and of how the counselor is called by God to minister truth and love to the couple.

If the couple rejects the counselor's advice either to separate and abstain from sexual intercourse or to marry, the couple also has a dilemma. Like all humans, their tendency will be to justify themselves and to rationalize their sin. They might defensively blame the counselor for being judgmental. If so, they will probably benefit little from future counseling. Or they might withdraw from future confrontation by not returning to counseling or by seeking another counselor. Or they might resist passively, ostensibly listening to the counselor but actually doing nothing that the counselor suggests.

The couple might also react to the confrontation in a non-defensive way. Usually, that involves perceiving the confrontation not as hostile but as loving—which can be aided by the way that the pastor confronts them. If the couple hears the message of the counselor without getting defensive, counseling can usually progress.

Preparing the Couple for Childbirth

There are several steps in preparing the cohabiting couple for childbirth. Rather than teaching them the mechanics of childbirth and delivery, you can refer them to one of the many classes offered by health care professionals concerning labor, delivery, and post-partum care. These classes might include information about pain control, such as the Lamaze or Bradley methods. Some classes offered through the local Red Cross usually focus less on pain control than on baby care and the health of the mother.

The counselor might help the couple maintain a vibrant relationship despite the changes required by the birth of the child. Research has consistently shown that having a child strains a marriage and results in a decline in satisfaction.[19] Usually, the birth is followed by a "baby honeymoon" in which the couple feel bonded closer.[20] As the pressures of (a) caring for an infant, (b) dealing with a change in intimacy between them, and (c) resolving conflicts inherent in the new decisions, they often grow apart. The counselor can alert them to the many potential changes and help them plan ways to handle the changes. (These changes are dealt with in more detail in the following chapter on birth of the first child early in marriage.)

The counselor can also help the couple decide whether they wish to begin their marriage together with a new infant or whether they want to place the child for adoption. It might be necessary for the counselor to recommend local agencies that handle adoptions and to help the couple work through the grief that they will experience when they give up their child. It is important to stress that though they feel pain at the loss, the child will likely be raised in a home that loves and accepts him or her. Adopting couples are carefully screened to insure that they provide an excellent home for the adopted child.

Preparing the Couple for Marriage

The couple who decide to keep their child and to marry will be piling two stressors on top of each other.[21] They will cope with a child better if they have been married for a while prior to its birth. Although marriage will be different for the couple who have cohabited than for the couple who have not cohabited, there will still be adjustments. The counselor usually has difficulty convincing the couple that their cohabiting experience has not fully prepared them for marriage. The counselor can describe the likely changes and discuss the belief of the couple that they will stay together as long as they love each other. Nonetheless, the couple will be unlikely to agree that marriage will change their relationship.

Commitment must be discussed at length with the cohabiting couple, but not to such length that they begin to pit commitment against love. Throughout the Bible love and commitment are not separated. The biblical norm is "You shall love the Lord your God with all your heart, and with all your soul, and with all your mind. This is the great and first commandment" (Matt. 22:37–38). This includes both commitment *and* emotional (heart) love. Marriage is, of course, God's metaphor for our relationship with him. Whenever we overstress commitment, people stop paying attention to how much love they feel for one another and soon the love erodes. Whenever we overstress love, people forget that they have taken vows for a lifetime of fidelity.

The *legal* bond of marriage changes the couple's relationship. It does not merely add a new dimension. It changes the nature of the relationship—in the minds of the couple, in the mind of society, and in the mind of God. Consequently, some of the relationship "rules" are likely to be renegotiated after cohabiting couples marry. This means that some conflict is likely soon after marriage. Counselors can help the couple work out the new rules of their marriage and deal with unanticipated changes in their relationship. Research on programs that prepare couples for marriage has shown that they have few long-term effects except when done a few months *after* the marriage.[22] I anticipate that the same will be true in preparing cohabiting couples for marriage. It is difficult for them to anticipate how married life will differ from cohabitation until they have experienced the differences.

Helping the Couple Cope with Abortion

Sadly, many cohabiting couples will elect to abort the baby prior to (and sometimes even after) consulting a counselor. Later, the couple has difficulty with guilt over their decision. The counselor is often asked to help absolve the couple from their guilt feelings. We can confidently announce to the couple that, "If we say we have no sin, we deceive ourselves and the truth is not in us. If we confess our sins, he is faithful and just, and will forgive our sins and cleanse us from all unrighteousness" (1 John 1:8–9).

If the couple confess and repent of their sin, they are forgiven. Despite the fact of forgiveness, though, they do not always feel forgiven. Often we attempt to comfort them by assuring them of the reliability and veracity of God's Word. Although this often helps, guilt feelings sometimes creep back. One reason this happens is because people have both a verbal and an imaginal part of their brain. The left hemisphere of their cortex thinks logically and verbally, while the right hemisphere thinks metaphorically, pictorially, and with dreams. When we appeal to the truth of Scripture, we involve only the left hemisphere of the brain. The woman's images of going through the abortion and the male partner's vicarious imagination can continue to haunt the couple. To effect full relief from the suffering of guilt over the abortion, the counselor can use a fantasy replay of the abortion in which the woman imagines Jesus meeting her. She can confess directly to him and can imagine his forgiveness directly. This adapts the method of inner healing recommended by many therapists and ministers to the guilt of abortion.[23]

Counseling Charles and Cathy

Having decided to keep their baby, Charles and Cathy quickly arranged a marriage by Pastor Bob. He came to their home at their request. After holding the baby and talking about the delivery and about how much they appreciated his visit to Cathy during her stay in the hospital, Charles and Cathy began to explore their future.

Charles: Pastor Bob, over the last week we have done lots of thinking and praying about our living situation. We have decided that we want to get married, and we wondered if you would perform the ceremony.

Pastor Bob: It's quite a responsibility having a new child, isn't it? Tell me how you have arrived at your decision to marry.

Cathy: Deciding to keep Angie was what got us thinking about it at first. We thought that it isn't fair to her to make her grow up with peers who won't understand that her parents aren't married.

Charles: There are a lot of other things that we talked about, too. We are tired of having people in the church look at us with accusation. They are very accepting for the most part, but some people don't understand that we love each other but just didn't feel quite ready for marriage.

Pastor Bob: But now you feel ready for marriage?

Charles: Now we're ready. We know it'll be hard. But we decided to keep Angie and to put up with the hardships.

Pastor Bob: You said that you didn't feel quite ready for marriage until now. Why did you not feel ready?

Cathy: I think I was ready, but Charles thought that we ought to get established in our careers before we decided for sure to commit to marriage.

Pastor Bob: But now it seems that you are even less settled in your careers and have more responsibilities than you did before Angie was conceived. What makes you feel you are ready now?

Charles: The birth made us see how much we really loved each other. We both wanted to do what would be best for the other—even though we thought we would each have trouble with it. I wanted to keep Angie but thought she would tie me down. So both of us said we would give up Angie. When we left Angie for adoption and went home, we talked and discovered that we both were laying down our wants for the other. We thought that would be a good foundation for marriage.

Pastor Bob: That is definitely what love is all about. I think you are right. That is a good foundation for marriage. But the best foundation is Jesus Christ. He wants you to give your whole lives to him and that will just multiply the love you have for each other.

Cathy: I want to have a marriage that is blessed by the Lord.

Charles: So do I.

Pastor Bob: That's great. What would it mean to you having a marriage that is blessed by the Lord?

Cathy: It would mean keeping him at the center of our marriage. And trying to live a life that is pleasing to him.

Pastor Bob: How about you, Charles? You have suddenly gotten quiet.

Charles: I guess I am realizing how selfish I have been and how stubborn. I remember how you talked to us earlier about our living together and about that not being in line with God's plan for our lives. I was pretty stubborn about that. We just ignored you, like we knew best. It is hard to admit it, but I have been pretty rebellious. I'm sorry.

Pastor Bob: Charles, I am sure that the Holy Spirit has been working with you to get you to this point.

Cathy: I've been callous about it, too.

Pastor Bob: It makes me feel good for you that you are about to restore your relationship with the Lord. There's one other thing that you might consider doing.

Cathy: What's that?

Pastor Bob: You might think about talking to the people during the Bible study group and telling them some of the things you have been thinking concerning your stubbornness or your rebelliousness and about your love for each other. I think that some of the people in the study have had a hard time understanding your cohabitation, and they might need to be involved in your forgiveness. You know, James tells us to ". . . confess your sins to one another, and pray for one another, that you may be healed" (James 5:16a). I think some healing is needed—not just in restoring you to full fellowship with the Lord, but also within the congregation.

Charles: I never thought about it before, but now I see that our sin was actually hurting others. Ouch. That really hurts.

Not every cohabiting couple makes such healing decisions. Pastor Bob kept the communication lines open and stayed true to his understanding of Scripture. The Holy Spirit faithfully ministered to Charles and Cathy, bringing them to the place of increased maturity and to confession—even public confession—and repentance.

PREVENTING COHABITATION

Prevention of cohabitation in children of Christian parents begins with the attitudes of the parents. If parents are convinced that cohabitation is in opposition to God's law, then it will be discussed as being a *moral* decision rather than as being a simple decision about lifestyle. Sex can be talked about within the family as being beautiful when used as God intended it—as part of marriage. For many parents, it is difficult to discuss issues such as sexual behavior with their children; however, accurate transmission of values from parents to children depends upon values being prominent in the home and also upon how values are discussed—how the parents explicitly treat such things rather than assume the children understand. Children will often distort ambiguous messages (and sometimes even clear messages) to fit their preexisting beliefs—called assimilation by Piaget. The parents' best defenses against such distortions are (1) to be explicit about their values and (2) to provide a home environment that is supportive and rules that are clearly defined yet fair.

Within the Congregation

Both laypeople and ministers can help stem the rising tide of cohabitation within the church. Probably the best ways to accomplish this are (a) to give a clear message from the pulpit about cohabitation as being against God's law, (b) to hold Sunday school and other study classes on contemporary issues in Christian living (see Appendix 2 for a list of recommended readings), and (c) to be clear about the joys and benefits of Christian marriage and until then about the benefits of chastity (see Table 4).

Benefits of Chastity Before Marriage

1. Chastity before marriage gives the couple the opportunity to get to know each other thoroughly. Understanding the mate is not confused by strong sexual feelings.
2. Chastity before marriage insures that no pregnancy will occur.
3. Chastity before marriage virtually insures that neither mate will have a sexually transmitted disease.
4. Chastity before marriage prevents comparison with earlier partners and yields an experience of intimacy that each mate is sure is only shared with the other and with no one else.
5. In the event of a break-up prior to marriage, the pain of rejection is lessened if the sexual bonding has not taken place.
6. God says don't have sexual intercourse before marriage (1 Thess. 4:3; Col. 3:5; 1 Cor. 6:13, 18; Matt. 15:19).
7. Early sex and sex with multiple partners increases the risk of sexual dysfunction.
8. Having sex prior to marriage increases the appetite for sex and thus "cheapens" the male/female sex encounter, whereas only chastity sets sex apart as special.
9. Chastity before marriage provides a witness to Christians and non-Christians that someone is willing to challenge in a practical way the hedonistic values of our day.

Table 4

One of the dangers in taking a strong stand against cohabitation within the congregation is judging couples who are already cohabiting. Cohabitation, like any sin, is wrong. But as Christians, our response to the sinner must still be love and acceptance of him or her as a person. The Holy Spirit convicts of sin, not the congregation.

Within Society

Cohabitation is a moral problem in society and is thus within the legitimate realm of social action. In Virginia during 1985, a law against cohabitation was challenged in the court on the grounds of the "right to privacy" in the bedroom, i.e., that consenting adults should be allowed to do whatever they wish in the privacy of their bedrooms. The judge overturned the law, and the decision was appealed to a higher court. Several Christian lawyers in Richmond compiled an *amicus curiae* brief that argued that the court had an interest in regulating some of the behaviors that occurred in privacy between consenting adults. On the basis of this brief and because of procedural faults in the case, the higher court overturned the judge's decision and upheld the law. Other cases without procedural difficulties are now being considered within the judicial system, so within a year or two this issue will probably reach the Supreme Court. In one recent decision the Supreme Court ruled that homosexual behavior between consenting adults within the bedroom was not protected under the Constitution, which may bear on the cohabitation decision when it reaches the Supreme Court.

Laws that prohibit cohabitation as illegal can be important in regulating the conduct of youth (and even adults). We know from Kohlberg's theorizing that stage 4 of moral reasoning involves adherence to law.[24] If cohabitation is *illegal,* many people in stage 4 will at least think hard before cohabiting. (The illegality of cohabitation should also affect those in stage 3, people who rely on authorities to justify moral behavior.)

The political, legal, and judicial arenas are legitimate areas for Christians to have an impact on society. It is no different in principle to impose a Christian morality on all people than to impose a secular (non-Christian) morality on all people *if the majority of people agree.* The political process is designed to allow people to compete for whose morality will govern society. Someone's morality will govern.

One danger of activism for Christians is that we will become convinced that we know *the* Christian position on every issue. Other Christians will take different positions. If we judge our brother and sister Christians for their different political positions, we might find ourselves correct on an issue but disobeying the law of love within the church. We need to stay humble and continue to love our brothers and sisters who believe in ways that we do not.

CHAPTER SIX

PREGNANT NEWLYWEDS

WE HAVE ALREADY DEALT WITH the *earliness* of a pregnancy—coming while the woman was a teen (either married or unmarried) and while the woman and man were cohabiting but unmarried. In this chapter and the next, the emphasis is on the *pregnancy* which is made more stressful by its earliness. In the present chapter, I will discuss parenthood in general and the transition to parenthood, which affects the individuals and the marriage relationship. With that foundation, I will examine the particular stressors resulting from a transition from a state of unmarriage to being married. Finally, I will discuss the difficulties of parenthood while still adjusting to marriage. In a sense, I am still adjusting to marriage after sixteen years of it. I am definitely still adjusting to parent-hood, even though my oldest daughter is ten. But most adjustment to these two transitions occurs within two years.

EFFECTS OF HAVING A CHILD ON EACH PARENT

There is something terribly mixed up about our modern culture. When I say, "the agony and the ecstasy," people usually think about Michelangelo. When I say, "the thrill of victory, the agony of defeat," people usually visualize a soccer player leaping for joy or a ski jumper careening into a crowd of spectators. What *I* am talking about, though, is parenthood. The thrill of victory. The agony of defeat.

Age and Level of Development of the Parents

Parenthood stimulates mixed feelings, exercising the full range of emotions. Parents experience pride, love, joy, fear, pain, sadness, confidence, and worry. One parental task is to cope with the variety of emotions inherent in parenthood. Obviously, people will differ in their intellectual ability to learn from mistakes (which child rearing allows us ample opportunity to make), their knowledge about child rearing, their emotional stability, their resources, the demands on their time, their social and emotional support systems, and the number of gray hairs they have when their first child is born.

One important factor in how people will react to pregnancy, childbirth, and child rearing is the age and developmental level of the parents at the time of the birth. Married couples can give birth from their teens through their forties. Most first births occur when couples are in their twenties. Couples in their twenties usually are dealing with different developmental issues than couples in their thirties. In their twenties, a man and wife are coping with autonomy and separation from the parents. They establish a household but are usually unable to earn much money since one or both of them are probably in their first career job. Because of their financial needs, they are often tied to their parents with economic strings. Usually, too, they might have lived at home or college before marriage and thus resided under the economic care of their parents.

Couples in their twenties have generally established a personal identity during their college years but, because they are in their first jobs, they often have little sense of professional identity. As they make decisions about their work and become a part of the community, they begin to balance the needs of the twenties—autonomy and relatedness—forging a balance that is unstable and usually plastic.

Couples in their thirties are also struggling. Generally, they have already separated from their parents and established a separate residence with financial independence. Their incomes have risen as they gained experience in their careers. If they lived alone through their twenties, they may have each saved enough money to be more financially secure. The big struggle of the thirties is against overcommitment. Career demands are usually heightened and people in this age bracket struggle to "make a mark" on the world. Every club, organization, or group to which they belong begins to look to them as leaders. Whereas the person in the early twenties feels engulfed by his or her parents, the thirty-year-olds feel engulfed by life's demands. They struggle to extricate themselves from overcommitment and to retain a sense of autonomy, while not totally foresaking relatedness.

People at each age react to the birth of a first child and to marriage differently. Of course, the tasks of people in their forties differ from those of twenty- or thirty-year-olds; but because most people marry and start their families before forty, that will not be covered.

Effects of Pregnancy

An expectant mother was asked what pregnancy was like. "You think it's all in your womb," she said, "and then you find out that your whole life is pregnant."[1] Pregnancy is a life-changing event. It affects the body, the psychology, and the marital relationship. Psychologically, pregnancy involves two experiences—the "physical pregnancy" and the "social pregnancy."

The "physical pregnancy" is arbitrarily divided into trimesters—three three-month periods. Usually these trimesters coincide with the physical feelings of the woman. For example, the first trimester is usually characterized by the nausea of morning sickness, which might happen anytime during the day and not just in the morning. Other physical symptoms of early pregnancy include frequent urination, fatigue (which ends shortly after the last child graduates and leaves home), and changes in the woman's body such as darkening of the nipples, appearance of a dark line on the abdomen, and perhaps stretch marks on the thighs or abdomen.

In the second trimester, the hormone balance changes and the woman usually feels happy, more energetic and emotionally stable. During the third trimester, she usually feels heavy from the growth of the baby, awkward, "fat," and emotionally prone to sudden changes in mood. For instance, when Kirby was pregnant with Christen (our first), she was attending a course in child development at the University of Missouri. In the middle of the class, she suddenly began to cry, for no apparent reason. The teacher, an experienced pro, checked to see whether something had precipitated the crying, and then merely informed the class, "Don't mind her. She's just pregnant. These things happen." Kirby continued to cry intermittently for about thirty minutes, then stopped for no apparent reason, and resumed normal operations. I asked her why she thought she had cried. "It seemed like the thing to do at the time," she said blandly.

The "social pregnancy" is often different from the physical pregnancy. The first stage of the social pregnancy generally begins when someone notices that the woman might be pregnant. Seiden-Miller divided pregnant women into three groups: true planners, sort-of-planners, and nonplanners.[2] The true planners, those who intentionally tried to get pregnant, usually noticed the changes in their bodies that signified the onset of pregnancy—missed period, nausea, or increased frequency of urination. They were quick to interpret their physical symptoms as pregnancy—quicker than the sort-of-planners and nonplanners. Most of the sort-of-planners (those who weren't really trying but who would not be disturbed if pregnancy occurred) and the nonplanners relied on physicians to interpret their symptoms as pregnancy. Some even went to the doctor without the slightest suspicion that they were pregnant. Today, ten years after

Seiden-Miller's study, more sort-of and nonplanners would probably diagnose their pregnancy using commercial pregnancy tests,[3] but they would still detect the pregnancy later than planners.

The second stage of social pregnancy occurs when the woman feels the baby move and when changes in the woman's body begin to be noticeable. Usually, a woman feels "definitely pregnant" at that time. She will schedule regular visits to the obstetrician, which continually remind her that she is definitely pregnant. Often, she will begin to wear pregnancy clothes during this time, even though her physical size may not require the loose-fitting clothing yet. Some of her friends look at her askance and remark, "You're definitely pregnant."

The third stage of social pregnancy is characterized by preoccupation with becoming a parent. Couples often attend classes to prepare them for childbirth; they redecorate the baby's room, secure baby clothes, pack their bag for the hospital visit, attend baby showers, talk about having babies with everyone they know, repack their bag for the hospital, and have regular false labors which allow them to speak with their obstetrician frequently—and check to see whether their bag is packed for the hospital.

Psychologically, the pregnancy has a strong impact on both mother- and father-to-be. She often feels fulfilled as a person. The transition to motherhood is sometimes seen as the most significant transition in the life of a woman.[4] Despite the feeling of fulfillment, though, most women have misgivings about their ability to be good mothers. These fears, anxieties, and feelings of fulfillment and confidence intermingle throughout pregnancy. Some studies have found that conflict over the upcoming birth is high early in pregnancy, tapering off later,[5] while other studies have found that conflict and ambivalence increased throughout pregnancy.[6] Probably the contradictory findings are due to studying two types of women. If the birth signifies a loss of work that the woman values and a perceived increase in responsibility that she does not want, she will likely experience increased turmoil as the due date approaches. If the birth of the child signifies a release from work that she finds unfulfilling or an opportunity to be a mother, which she values, then she will likely experience decreased turmoil as the due date approaches.

Fathers-to-be might have similar mixed feelings about the impending birth of the child. On one hand, they feel proud of their virility. Bill Cosby points out, "Even if [the new father] is afraid of garter snakes, he feels positively heroic [at having made his wife pregnant]."[7] On the other hand, he wonders whether he will be a good father and whether the presence of the child will affect his marriage.[8]

Effects of Preparation for Childbirth

In the 1980s and beyond (I trust), the effect of childbirth on parents cannot be considered apart from the many classes that prepare couples for childbirth. It has become commonplace for couples to attend either Red Cross-sponsored childbirth classes or a class that stresses pain control during labor and delivery—such as Lamaze or Bradley. During the years when our four children were born, I investigated the effectiveness of many parts of the Lamaze method of pain control. In a series of experiments, I showed that patterned breathing, attention to focal points, rehearsal of the techniques, and especially husband coaching (a) were important in reducing perceptions of pain and distress and (b) were associated with fewer requests for medication and with medication being requested later in labor.[9] Effleurage (gentle self-massage) was not effective at relieving pain, and in fact resulted in increased pain.[10]

Great claims have been made for the benefits of the Lamaze method—including painless childbirth. Research shows that the Lamaze method can reduce perceived pain but not eliminate it. These classes have an important social function for many couples. They provide a structured interaction each week before, during, and after the classes. They also provide activities around which the couple can interact between classes, such as practicing their pain control techniques together. Finally, they provide a stimulus to discuss the baby and its effects on their lives. Markman and Kadushin have shown that attending Lamaze classes has resulted in improved marital satisfaction.[11]

Sometimes I wonder, though. Can we really prepare a couple

for childbirth? Perhaps we should broaden our horizons. Someone should develop classes that prepare couples for what they will encounter in Lamaze classes. I'm not talking about the movies about childbirth that must be watched. I'm talking about the personality transformation that occurs in the father-to-be as a result of these classes. You think I'm joking? Just listen.

In one Lamaze class that Kirby and I attended, there were twenty couples. I watched one night as they entered the hospital lobby—each husband with his wife's pillow tucked under his arm. Now *that's* chivalrous. Wives were breathing regularly, "Heh, heh, heh." They were practicing their breathing exercises, which they forgot to practice during the week. Periodically the husbands made some virile-sounding comment, such as, "Okay, honey, let's do choo-choo breathing now." Or, "How about some hoo-ha breathing, sweetie?"

Discussing "choo-choo breathing" in public *requires* preparation.

Lamaze classes stress tenderness, warmth, and support as the manly qualities that they are. Clint Eastwood dialogue is discouraged. Empathy is rewarded.

Some husbands even need to learn to cope with *couvade.* Couvade is a cultural phenomenon, rarely practiced in contemporary United States settings. In couvade, the woman in labor goes into the field, squats, and has her baby with little more than a grimace. The husband takes to the bed and apparently feels extreme pain, moaning and writhing. (It's a dirty job, but someone has to do it.) It is the ultimate in empathy.

There was one man in our Lamaze class who apparently experienced couvade. He woke up, dressed, and went to work. About ten o'clock, he began to have great pain in his abdomen. He called his wife, "Honey, I'm in labor. Is our baby coming?"

"No, dear."

"But I'm in enormous pain. Don't tell me it's false labor," he said.

"I wouldn't do that. But this morning, you wore our ten-year-old's undershorts to work."

That ended the couvade.

Effects of Childbirth

Like pregnancy, childbirth happens in stages, too.[12] Caesarean births involve about 18 percent of all births[13] and involve different stages than unassisted births.[14] For unassisted births, the beginning of childbirth is *labor*. The onset of labor is a social phenomenon. I know it *feels* like a physical phenomenon, but *someone* must define the woman as officially in labor. In many cases it is the hospital staff, who base their judgment on the dilation of the woman's cervix and on the apparent strength and regularity of the woman's contractions. In other cases, the woman defines herself as in labor, usually phoning the physician and alerting him. The onset of labor signifies focused attention on the birth. Normal schedules are abandoned and the woman is either hospitalized or remains at home, where she closely monitors the progress of labor by timing the duration of and intervals between contractions. Often the husband is involved in monitoring the contractions.

As the length and strength of contractions increase, the couple which has prepared for childbirth will use its Lamaze breathing patterns. In the early stages of labor, there is excitement. As the discomfort increases, the wife can be more blunt and less considerate of her husband's more tender sensibilities. "Don't touch me," she might yell in one breath. Then she could shriek at the hospital staff, "Come and knock me out and just take the baby." During the later stages of labor, the wife's wounding words are usually considered a product of her pain and are not taken too seriously. The last stage of labor is called "transition." I first had difficulty determining what the transition was from and to. Then I decided it was a personality transition in the wife. I only discovered later that it was transition to the second stage of childbirth.

The second stage of childbirth is *parturition*. It begins when the hospital staff or physician determines that the cervix is fully dilated and effaced and birth is therefore imminent. Parturition ends with the delivery of the child. Generally, in the hospital the wife will be moved from the labor room to the delivery room at parturition.

Kovit has defined three substages of parturition: patient introduction, baby announcement, and "I'm done—Congratulations."[15] The patient introduction substage involves the trip to the delivery room and the introductions of the mother to the delivery personnel.

"Good evening, Mrs. Smith. I'm Doctor Jones. I'll be attending. . . . What's that?"

"Aarrgghh."

"Oh, yes, by all means, do push. Let me introduce to you Doctor Franks. She's our anesthesiologist. And this is. . . ."

Obviously some of the social chitchat is not fully appreciated by the woman. The staff usually assures the woman that the worst part is over.

The baby announcement substage usually begins with a sighting of the baby's head, which is announced with the gusto of a sailor spotting land after being lost at sea for a month. That encourages the woman to persevere and ultimately brings about the announcement of the sex of the child. At last, the piercing cry of the child simultaneously announces the functioning of the infant's lungs and the beginning of sleep-interrupted nights for the couple over the upcoming months. The baby's physical condition is assessed, and the physician usually finishes by delivering the placenta and suturing any tears or surgical cuts during delivery. At the conclusion, congratulations are given on the child, ending the parturition stage of delivery.

The third stage of childbirth is *postpartum*. Generally, this refers to the period of birth of the child until the woman's body has returned roughly to the prepregnancy state. Most doctors claim six to eight weeks as the duration of the postpartum stage. Often hospitals will allow the mother to hold and even nurse the baby on the delivery table. Most hospitals allow the parents to hold the baby in the recovery room once the baby has been cleaned. "Rooming in," which involves having the mother and infant in the same room during the stay in the hospital, is less common, but usually the mother can have the child in her room whenever she wishes.

Recovery at home is facilitated by support systems. The new grandparents often visit and provide assistance while the new mother is recovering. Church communities also often assist through preparing meals and doing other chores for the new parents.

Effect of Being the Parent of an Infant

Being the parent of an infant involves the sensitivity of an "empath," the frustration tolerance of a New York cabbie, and the constitution of an Iron Man Triathlon contestant. Millions do it yearly, and survive. But not without having the new child transform their lives.

One of the first ways the infant changes things is by affecting the parents' private time. True, no human infant has the power to subtract time from the life of the parent. It just seems that way. The infant is lying peaceably in the crib, cooing and discussing the color of his or her room with the stuffed animal which shares the crib. Suddenly, the infant realizes that something is terribly wrong. Life is horrible. The world is ending. Pain rifles his or her body. The only solution for this terrible problem is to announce the calamity to the world. Loudly.

The world in this case consists of one naked, warm mother, who intends to relax for a moment in a warm tub. The instant before the catastrophe she slipped silently into the tub. When the infant calls, though, Mother answers. Leaping from the tub, she sloshes water onto the rug. As she jerks the towel from the rack, she upsets a container of after-bath powder onto the now-damp, previously-clean carpet in the bathroom. Undaunted, she runs toward the baby's room, hitting the doorway and bruising her elbow en route. Just as she enters the baby's room, the infant squirms and says, "Burp." Then, silence.

"It wouldn't have been so bad if you had gone, 'BURP' or even if you had let me pat you and then burped," she tells the infant. "But no—all by yourself, you go 'burp.'"

This scene, with some variations, is acted out hundreds of times each day. I know mothers who talk to themselves. They swear that the baby has a television monitoring system in his or her room that alerts the baby whenever the mother is about to have a moment to herself. In her less frustrated moments, the mother knows that the baby does not wet, have messy diapers, get hungry, get sleepy, or simply need to burp intentionally. In fact, the lack of intentionality of the baby's actions means that the parent must be available to the baby whenever he or she has a need. Determining whether the baby's need or the parent's need is stronger is difficult and creates numerous opportunities for internal conflict in the mother. "I have no time for myself anymore" is the common lament of the new parent.

Parents must care directly for or insure the care of their infant constantly. This is the second way the parents' lives are affected. They must curtail many of their activities, or at best modify them to include the infant, the payment of a babysitter, or a visit with the infant's grandparents.

Thirdly, the baby changes his or her parents by filling an affectional need. Both women and men generally express affection for their children, though this has not always been true historically.[16] LaRossa has argued that the affection parents feel for their children depends on the value they place on their children relative to other activities.[17] He wonders what the effects of our individualistic and career-oriented society will be on future childrearing attitudes and practices.

There are at least a thousand other ways that having a child changes parents' lives. Let me mention only a couple of the most important.

Childbirth changes the parents' wardrobe. Each day the parent is burped on (necessitating three changes of shirts and one change of pants), spilled on (one complete change), and wet on (which the parent decides merely to wash out and live with). After six months, the original wardrobe is completely worn out, faded and frayed from repeated washings. The new parent decides to buy a new wardrobe. Multicolored. Paisleys. Checks and plaids—prefaded. One pair of camouflage combat fatigues for wearing around the house when one is certain to meet no one.

Second, being a parent changes eating habits. At the table, the parent instinctively eats with one hand and feeds someone else with the other hand. Sometimes a parent finds that while changing the baby's diapers, talking to the baby, washing clothes (the baby's and her own), and maintaining a household, she missed lunch. Perhaps the child is too hot, too cold, too wet, too hungry, or too sleepy. Perhaps he or she is disturbed by the combat fatigues, which haven't been changed for three days.

Nietzsche said, "That which does not kill me makes me stronger." But then Nietzsche was a philosopher, not a parent. What did he know? Every parent knows "that which does not kill me makes me *grayer.*" But, in getting grayer, presumably parents become wiser and more capable of love. They demonstrate daily what agape love really is—laying down their lives for someone else. They see the toll that agape love takes, and in their reflective moments they praise God for his grace and wisdom in making them parents.

EFFECTS OF HAVING A CHILD ON THE MARRIAGE RELATIONSHIP

Effect on Marital Satisfaction

Becoming a parent, or even conceiving a child, has an impact on the couple's marital satisfaction. In a study of Lutherans,[18] about one thousand families were surveyed at different points in the family life cycle. The researchers measured the couples' overall quality of life, their family life satisfaction, and their marital satisfaction. Neither quality of life nor family satisfaction changed across the family life cycle. However, marriage satisfaction changed according to which phase of life the participants were in. Marriage satisfaction was highest prior to having children and after retirement, when all the children were gone from the home.

Beverley Buston and I have reviewed the effects of the transition to parenthood on the marriage relationship using theoretical writings and eighty-four empirical studies.[19] Let me summarize the results and refer the reader to the review paper for the documentation of each point.

1. In direct comparisons, childless couples have been found to be happier with their relationships than couples with children (nine supporting studies).

2. Other studies have compared couples at different stages of the family life cycle. In stages where children are not in the home, couples are generally more satisfied with their

marriages than in stages when children are in the home (nine supporting studies).

3. Marriage satisfaction has been found to be related inversely to the number of children that a couple has (five supporting studies, one study not supporting).

4. In experimental designs in which husbands and wives were tested before they gave birth and then again after they gave birth, the results were similar. There is a period of increased marriage satisfaction shortly after the birth called the "baby honeymoon" (three supporting studies, one study not supporting), which is followed by a decline in marriage satisfaction to a level below the prebirth level (twelve supporting studies).

5. Some examples of positive effects of childbirth on the parents' marriage relationship have been reported, but these have generally been weak (nine supporting studies).

6. Most research has found that becoming a parent is more stressful for the mother than for the father (thirteen supporting studies). For example, Harriman (1983) found that wives perceived more change in their personal lives but husbands perceived more change in their marital and sexual lives.

7. The child can affect the parents' relationship, but the parents' relationship can also affect the behavior of the child (two supporting studies).

8. The extent and type of impact of the child on the marriage often depends on whether the child was wanted or planned, and on whether many of the parents' expectations about childbirth and child rearing are violated (two supporting studies).

9. The effect of the child on the marriage extends throughout the entire life of the parents. For example, Myers-Walls identified five areas of impact: work, social life, marriage, housekeeping, and childrearing.[20] Harriman identified no less than twenty-one areas of impact. Among those were twelve personal areas and six marital areas.[21]

As can be seen from this simple "box score" approach, having children usually affects the marriage relationship in a negative way. Generally, when a study did not support a finding it usually indicated that no effect was found, and not that the opposite effect was found.

146

Effect on Time Schedules

Marital satisfaction is affected by having children because other aspects of marriage are affected, notably time schedules and conflict over relationship rules—which affect couples involved in ongoing power struggles more than those couples not engaged in ongoing power struggles.

As I have argued in chapter 2, having children forces couples to change their time commitments. Nine independent studies on the transition to parenthood support that argument.[22] Individuals differ in how much their time schedules are disrupted and in how they perceive the new schedule relative to the prebirth schedule. Usually, the greater the disruption the more negatively the person perceives the change.

Nor does the effect of childbirth on the couple's time commitments occur only after birth. Usually, the pregnancy begins to change the lives of the new parents-to-be. Initially, expectant parents report more intimacy in their marriages. They say they are more connected and emotionally closer to one another.[23] They say that the later stages of pregnancy provide them with a common focus to their marriage and they often do new activities together, such as attend preparation for childbirth classes and do housework that is concerned with the child's space. The visible evidence of pregnancy is viewed as a tangible expression of the love of the couple for each other. Even though couples say their relationship is improved by pregnancy, most couples report that their sexual relationship suffers during pregnancy. In the last trimester, sexual relations generally fall off in frequency for a variety of reasons.[24] LaRossa found that if he asked couples *if* their sex lives had changed during pregnancy, almost all couples gave reasons *why* it had *decreased*.[25]

In addition, during pregnancy the man and woman often relate to each other differently around the house. The husband is often more solicitous to the wife than before.[26] Usually there are some alterations in the way that housework is allocated. For example, during pregnancy the husband tends to help the wife with some of the more traditionally "feminine" household duties, but after the birth the husband and wife interact in more "traditional" roles in dividing household tasks. Several studies have suggested that division of household tasks becomes more traditional after the birth of the first child,[27] but the "traditionality" of the division of labor generally depends on when the measurements are made.[28]

Change in time allocation implies that the couple have adopted new roles. Research on "role strain theory" is voluminous.[29] Most new parents feel conflict among their many new roles.[30] For instance, an entire body of research investigates the conflicts mothers face between work and motherhood roles. The most common complaint of new parents is that there is not enough time to meet all the demands, such as taking care of the baby, managing their relationship with each other, handling work and household responsibilities, maintaining friendships, and getting enough relaxation and (especially) sleep. Parents cope with role strain in a number of ways. (1) They might seek and use information. The information is obtained from child rearing newsletters, television, books, friends, relatives, counselors, Sunday school classes, and other helpful people. (2) They redefine their situation as positive instead of negative. For example, the husband and wife might think how their increased life demands demonstrate love for their child. (3) They handle role strain by setting priorities. Some activities are eliminated or drastically reduced, such as having a moment to oneself. (4) Some couples handle role strain through increased attention to family planning. After the new child comes, birth-control methods might be scrupulously observed and the couple might decide to change its opinion of the optimal spacing between children (or optimal number of children). (5) Couples might cope with role strain by seeking help from professionals or other knowledgeable people. (6) Couples might cope with role strain by arranging support groups. In our church, many of the couples were in their childbearing years simultaneously. Kathy White, helped by several other mothers, began a support-and-information group for mothers called "Motherhood as a Career." Each month, they invited a knowledgeable person to speak to the group about some aspect of childrearing. In addition, the regular meetings provided a source of support and commonality that bonded the women together emotionally.

Changes in time schedules can also disrupt the balance among distancing, coacting, and intimacy-producing activities. Numerous researchers have linked intimacy to marital satisfaction.[31]

The effects of pregnancy and childbirth on the marriage relationship change over time. Generally, despite the decrease in sexual activity during the last part of pregnancy, they feel more intimate during pregnancy and shortly after the birth of the child, but as they adjust to the presence of the child in the home, they begin to feel a loss of intimacy and a decrease in marital satisfaction.

Effect on Conflict

Despite the feelings of increased intimacy during the pregnancy, couples often experience substantial conflict during that time.[32] The amount of conflict depends on both "ideology" and "dependence."[33] Ideology refers to the beliefs of each partner about how power should be distributed within the relationship. Their agreement or disagreement in beliefs is generally more important than what the beliefs are. For instance, when both believe that the man is the head of the household, they will likely experience little conflict; similarly if they both believe that the household should be run by the mother. On the other hand, a husband and wife who differ in beliefs will experience conflict regardless of the individual beliefs.

Dependence refers to the psychological need people have for each other. Dependence has less to do with what people say about themselves than with how they act. Furthermore, dependence is a characteristic of two people within a specific relationship, not the characteristic of a person. If one spouse is more dependent on the other spouse than vice versa, conflict will usually be resolved in the favor of the less dependent spouse. This might or might not result in tension in the relationship. The more dependent spouse might feel that he or she is deriving what is desired from the relationship and is thus willing to give up some power in return. Conflict occurs when the partners feel that they are not receiving equitably in relation to what they are giving.

149

During pregnancy many occurrences might change the balance of power between the spouses. For example, if they held differing opinions about the woman's role as a career woman, they might find that they begin to agree about her role when she stops work because of the pregnancy. On the other hand, in a different couple the woman might lose power in the relationship because she stops providing financial resources to the marriage. One sobering statistic indicates the extent of power struggles in some marriages during pregnancy: the wife is more likely to be abused physically during pregnancy than prior to pregnancy.[34]

Conflict increases not just in pregnancy but also after childbirth.[35] Perhaps the main reason for increased conflict is that pregnancy and (especially) the postchildbirth period provide numerous occasions for the couple to disagree over the decisions they must make. During pregnancy, some couples anticipate the decisions required in childbirth and begin then to work out their differences. For other couples, the birth brings disagreements to the forefront. The period shortly after the birth of the child—the "baby honeymoon"—serves as an emotional buffer between the pregnancy and the period of hard decision-making. In addition, many issues that had supposedly been resolved through discussion during pregnancy are different when they are actually faced. For example, one well-informed couple realized how physically draining the birth would likely be for the mother. They had discussed the additional chores that would be necessary for harmonious rearing of the infant. However, when the birth came, the husband was reluctant to change diapers, which he had easily agreed to do prior to the birth. Furthermore, the mother was more "protective" of the infant than she thought she would be, so she tended to resist having the father handle the child as much as they had agreed to do during the pregnancy.

Summary and Look Ahead

Clearly, the transition to parenthood—from pregnancy to the postdelivery adjustment—has an enormous effect on most married couples. It affects the spouses individually and it affects the marriage relationship by affecting the time

150

commitments, roles, intimacy, and conflict patterns. By itself, becoming parents can be extremely stressful; however, when the stress of the transition to parenthood is added to other stresses—such as the transition to marriage (in this chapter), the adjustment to an earlier recent birth (chapter 7), the realization that the new child is "one too many" (chapter 8), the onset of menopause (chapter 9), and the difficulty of coping with a child who is difficult, deformed, retarded, or chronically ill (chapter 10)—the stress can be overwhelming.

THE STRESS OF THE TRANSITION TO MARRIAGE

By the time a man and woman marry, they have usually spent time together, time characterized by activities that are coactive and intimate. As their relationship progresses, generally, the intimacy increases—not just the sexual intimacy they share but other intimate activities as well. They spend time planning the honeymoon and talking about what they value. They discuss whatever is important to them and try to resolve differences in their values. Time not spent in discussions that make the self more transparent to the future spouse is generally spent doing pleasant activities together. They might go to the mountains together, play tennis, attend parties with friends, and generally structure much of their "free time" doing activities jointly.

Of course, all people have a need for aloneness or distance as well as needs for coaction and intimacy. The need for distance is met by simply going home. Perhaps the engaged couple will spend twenty-five hours together during a week. Of that, ten is spent in intimacy-producing conversation or other activity and fourteen is spent in coactivity. Only one hour is spent in each other's presence engaging in distancing activities.

However, immediately after the couple returns from the honeymoon, their time schedules change dramatically. Each arises and, after a warm kiss, they trot off to their separate activities. He reads the paper, showers, shaves, and prepares for work. She prepares her daily lessons and studies for a test in one of her college classes. They eat breakfast preoccupied by the events likely to occur in the day.

When she comes home from school in the afternoon no one

is home, so she studies alone, and then begins dinner. He arrives later and they eat together and have a pleasant afternoon playing tennis and an enjoyable night watching television and making love. Over the course of a few months, the couple might notice that a subtle change has occurred in their relationship. Now, they spend fifty hours together each week. However, thirteen are spent in intimacy-producing activities, eighteen in coactivity, but nineteen are spent in distancing activities. The wife begins to feel, "The romance is going out of our relationship. Before we married, he never used to read the paper and just ignore me." Actually, he did. He read the paper each morning when he was home alone. But because of the different *balance* of intimacy, coaction, and distance, it feels to the wife like the romance is going out of the relationship.

One additional change makes it difficult to adjust to marriage. The attributions of why the couple is together—because they love each other or because they are legally married—change merely because the couple marries.

Adjustment to Marriage

Marriage requires certain tasks of the newly wedded couple. They must establish an independent household and separate emotionally and financially from their parents. Because the couple is often financially needy, separation from parents can sometimes be difficult. Relationships with in-laws can be complicated by proximity and the maintenance of financial ties.

Establishing a viable sexual relationship can be difficult, too. For the man and woman who are both virgins at marriage, the change in status from sex as forbidden fruit to sex as sumptuous feast is gradual. They must learn how to make love in ways that satisfy both partners and must overcome longstanding prohibitions and inhibitions. If they have sexual experiences that are unsatisfying or acrimonious early in their marriage, they can quickly become locked into unsatisfying sexual relationships.

For couples in which one or both partners have had sexual experience prior to marriage, the transition from illegitimate to legitimate sexual relations can sometimes inhibit them. If the spouses have had sexual experience with a partner other than the new spouse, the tendency to compare lovers can often be a stumbling block to a good sexual relationship. Some people report "flashbacks" to lovemaking episodes with earlier lovers which inhibit them from developing a satisfying sexual relationship with their spouse.

The early part of marriage is generally characterized by a "honeymoon" which is distinct from the one-week honeymoon traditionally taken just after the marriage. This "honeymoon" may last anywhere from one and a-half minutes to one and a-half years after the marriage ceremony. During that period, each spouse encounters violations by the other spouse of the expected "rules" of marriage.

For example, Sue and Bob have been married two weeks. Sue casually says to Bob, "Bob, lambchop, darling (or something equally as romantic), how about taking the trash out, sweetie pie."

He smiles and says, "Sure, dumpling"; however, this is *not* what is going on in his mind. In his family of origin, taking out the trash was always woman's work. To him, it is an unnatural act for the man to take out the garbage. But he bites his tongue, smiles and, with his eyes glazed over, agrees to the onerous task. During the "honeymoon," both spouses will put aside their personal ideas about what the "right" marriage behavior is and accede to their spouse's wishes. Eventually, though, the "honeymoon" is over, and the spouse, when asked to do something not in line with his or her expectations, will object—sometimes loudly. Disagreements begin to erupt like initial tremors around Mount St. Helens. Before long, the couple is having a relatively high number of disagreements, especially when compared to the "honeymoon."

Although they do not like these disagreements, they are necessary to a good marriage. I examined marriages at three points in the family life cycle: married 0–3 years, 4–16 years, and 17–56 years.[36] I divided the marriages into those high in marital satisfaction and those low in marital satisfaction. For couples married from 0–3 years, those with happy marriages reported *more* minor disagreements than those with less happy marriages. Those with happy marriages were also *less* critical to themselves of their spouse than those with unhappy marriages. On the other hand, for couples married from 4–16 years and from 17–56 years, happy couples reported fewer disagreements and less criticism of their spouse than couples with less happy marriages. I concluded that early in marriage it is helpful for couples to have disagreements *if* they can resolve them. It prevents the build-up of resentment and criticism of their spouse. The newly wedded couple, once the "honeymoon" is complete, must move from having expectations on the basis of their family of origin to having expectations that have resulted from working out disagreements with the spouse.

PILING UP STRESSORS

When Holmes and Rahe examined stressful life events,[37] they found a "threshold" for stress in many people. Taking an empirical approach, they assigned "life change points" to stressful life events. They found that when a person had accumulated high amounts of life change points, the person became at risk for serious accidents and illnesses in the near future. For example, they found that people with 200–299 life change points had a better than 50 percent chance of an accident or illness within the next two years. People with 300 or more life change points had a better than 80 percent chance for an accident or illness. This suggests that there might be thresholds for how well people manage stress. As stressors build up, the person copes well with each additional stressor. Finally, though, the tolerance level is reached and the person's coping skills break down, being no longer capable of handling the stress. Something "snaps!"

McCubbin and Patterson suggested that families encounter stressors and used coping skills and resources in the same way as individuals.[38] The addition of the stressors of childbirth to the stressors of adjusting to being newly married might overtax the coping capabilities of some couples. Like many transitions, both marriage and parenthood place stress on the same parts of the relationship—time schedules (with the threat to established roles and intimacy-distance patterns) and disagreements. Because the stressors are in the same areas, the strains are not simply additive. Rather, the strains tend to be synergistic— that is, they produce effects that are greater than the sum of the components.

The issues about which couples disagree as they are adjusting to marriage are also similar to those about which couples disagree when they are adjusting to parenthood. Finances are troublesome in both instances. For example, when couples marry they are generally young enough so that they are in their first job within their career field. Their financial status is often tentative and they might even depend on one or both sets of in-laws for making ends meet. Having a child within a year or so of the marriage might greatly affect the financial status of the couple. The wife might take leave from work while she adjusts to the new child, or she might even stop work until the child is older (or she might never go back to work). In addition, the financial strain of having a baby and of supporting an infant will place additional financial burdens on the couple and will make them attend more closely to financial decisions. LaRossa has shown that people pay more attention to decision-making in an economy of scarcity than in an economy of plenty.[39] This is true whether the economy is monetary or involves the use of time.

Besides financial issues, the couple must deal with disruptions in their sexual relationship. Just as they are beginning to establish themselves, a pregnancy causes sexual difficulties, especially—as we have seen—in the final trimester.

Emotional stability, too, is affected by both marriage and pregnancy. In marriage, the unique rules of a marriage relationship must be negotiated, with the spouses beginning from the different rules they inherited from their families of origin. In pregnancy, the woman's hormonal variations often result in emotional swings.

One of the biggest tasks of marriage is to resolve issues of intimacy and dependency. The married couple must break away from the family of origin and establish their own intimacy and mutual dependence. Just as they begin to accomplish this, an early pregnancy and birth can renew issues of dependency because the infant is totally dependent on the new parents. If the husband and wife are struggling to be free from dependency on their own parents, this can raise serious conflicts both psychologically within each partner and socially within their relationship. In addition, as they establish patterns of intimacy and accept necessary distancing in their relationship, a new child will often make time demands that impair the tenuous patterns of intimacy.

Finally, couples early in marriage must disagree in order to form a solid relationship. Yet, after the "honeymoon" stage, adding pregnancy and the birth of an infant to ordinary marital disagreements contributes to the instability of the early marriage.

Overall, the couple who become pregnant early after their marriage are probably in for a difficult time as they try to adjust to two transitions. Conflict will usually be high and the couple will also generally have some difficulty with intimacy.

COUNSELING PREGNANT NEWLYWEDS

Although many of these couples are at risk for marital problems and for stress-related individual difficulties, most will handle their relationship strains with minimal intervention. Generally, the professional will serve merely as referral agent for those couples. They might be referred to preparation for childbirth classes, which serve as support groups in which couples can discuss their difficulties with other couples who are experiencing similar difficulties. In many groups, information about childbirth and parenting is less important than social support and the opportunity for the couple to interact around the birth of the child.

Church-related groups provide another source of social support and information. One difficulty of church-related groups is that sometimes too few people are near the same stage of life for the group to function effectively as a support. Other support can be derived from Bible study, prayer, or fellowship groups that are accepting and interested in the couple and their struggles. In fact, there is some benefit to having groups with couples at different life stages.

In a study of marriage enrichment groups, Worthington, Buston, and Hammonds[40] found that the information imparted was less valuable than the social support. The effects of the group were not entirely positive. Some treatments that provided information necessary to improve marriage actually resulted in a decrease in intimacy in the couples. We hypothesized that the group took valuable time from the couple's week without allowing the couple extra time to interact intimately with each other. Those couples reported decreases in intimacy throughout treatment. The implication is that a highly structured group—such as a structured Bible study—might reduce a couple's intimacy rather than increase it. Presumably the individual's knowledge of the Bible and the application of biblical truths to his or her life might be strengthened, but the couple's marital intimacy would probably not be aided. The professional should understand the needs of the couple and the format of the group before recommending a group to the couple.

Another way that the professional can help the newly married couple who are pregnant is by providing information about the stresses and strains of the two transitions (for a list of some recommended readings, see Appendix 3).

For couples who are troubled and whose relationship is in danger, counseling might be appropriate. The counselor must assess the relationship thoroughly. Special attention must be paid to the way a couple uses its time and to the past and present patterns of intimacy. The counselor will try to assess the ways the man and woman have been affected by the transitions. The ways that they discuss their differences can be assessed through having them talk about a difference of opinion while being audiotaped. The types and topics of conflict must be identified.

After the intimacy and conflictual styles and topics are assessed, the counselor can recommend how counseling might proceed. The recommendation should include: (1) a conceptualization of the problem, (2) a recognition about how the recent transitions have affected the relationship, (3) a proposal about the goals for counseling—which will include helping the marriage become more intimate and helping the couple manage their disagreements more satisfactorily, (4) a rough idea of how the goals will be achieved, and (5) an approximation of how long the counseling should take.

Counseling should involve two major phases—breaking up old patterns of behavior and building new patterns. The counselor should tailor the treatment to the specific needs of the couple. For some, disruption in their intimacy will receive the most attention. For others, conflict management will be most time consuming. Generally, it is better to work on a few issues in counseling such as finances or sexual behavior or in-laws even though the man and woman present many issues that disturb them.

Once a single issue has been resolved, the themes of counseling should be clear. A second issue can then be broached and worked through. Generally, each problematic issue will involve similar themes. When they have worked through two or three issues, they should attempt to work on their problems without continuing counseling. If they are unable to resolve their problems without undue difficulty, counseling might resume and deal with a few additional issues. A complete account of my methods and theories for marriage counseling with Christian couples is given in the book *Counseling Married Christian Couples*.[41]

PREVENTION

Very few couples intentionally set out to become pregnant soon after their wedding. Generally, couples who achieve this feat do so despite their taking precautions with birth-control methods. Little can be done to prevent the problem. Most people realize that children place additional strains on their marriage. Generally, young couples might have unreasonable expectations that children might help a troubled marriage. If you are counseling a young couple prior to marriage, check out their assumptions about children and encourage them to put off having children until their marriage is well off the ground.

Even if they do become pregnant soon after the wedding, some preventive counseling is possible. You can counsel the couple about how to cope with the build-up of stressors during and after the pregnancy. Some of these methods include compartmentalization and compromise of standards.[42] Compartmentalization involves forgetting one role and the demands associated with that role while performing another role. For instance, the woman might concentrate on the caretaking functions while she is caring for the baby, but when the baby is asleep and the woman is at home with her husband, she gives him her full attention. Compromise of standards involves changing one's ideas about the level of performance to expect from oneself. For example, a woman who holds an ideal for herself as an immaculate housekeeper might change her standards when she finds that they conflict with spending adequate time with her baby and husband.

Other useful, natural coping strategies include flexibility, adaptability, and being more organized.[43] Given the usual infant, flexibility and adaptability come more easily than organization. The infant forces flexibility on the parent. You have plans. Tough. The kid has decided to be ill tonight. Besides that, the babysitter broke out in a rash today. Either you adapt to the changing situations and take the child with you to the company's formal dinner, or you remain flexible in your plans about going to the dinner at all. Being more organized when one has a baby is practically a *non sequitur.* Babies are the proof of the second law of thermodynamics, which (stated informally) is "in life, chaos increases." Worthington's corollary is "a parent always puts more energy into dressing children than they put into messing."

CHAPTER SEVEN

BACK-TO-BACK CHILDREN

COPING WITH A PREGNANCY, childbirth, and then an infant is one thing. Coping with two in rapid succession adds a new dimension to the word coping. When the close-together children come in a package labeled twins, count on overwhelmed parents. In chapter 6, I outlined the stresses and strains of the transition to parenthood. When that transition is followed immediately by a second birth, the effect is often magnified. In addition, children who follow other children very closely often do more than repeat the difficulties (and joys); they intensify them.

PREPARING FOR TWINS

Labor is proceeding on schedule. The woman is moved quickly to the delivery room. After seemingly countless pushes, a baby girl is delivered. As the nurses and physicians attend to the baby, one of the nurses glances at the mother. "You can stop pushing now, honey. It's all over."

"Nope," she strains.

"What do you mean 'nope'?"

"I can't stop pushing."

"Doctor Smith, I think there's someone who needs to see you," says the nurse. "She's coming out right now."

Husband swallows chewing gum. Doctor hustles over and does shortshop routine: Mama to Doc to nurse for a double play. After the doctor passes the second child to the nurse, he palpitates the woman's abdomen. "Anybody else at home in there?" he calls.

The first reaction of the parents when they discover at the delivery that they are blessed with twins is shocked disbelief, rapidly turning to shocked belief. Often the mother will simply want the birth to be finished, having just negotiated a long, hard labor. Usually, the father is happy and is often more involved in the birth of twins than he is in the birth of single children. "I grinned from heir to heir," one father crowed.

Shock and negative reactions can also occur. For example, if the parents had felt financially stressed with one birth, the thought of two births can be frightening. Or if the parents had their heart set on having a boy because of their three girls at home, and instead they had two more girls, usually the parents require a few days to be philosophical about the new developments.

Probably the largest shock of having unexpected twins is that the couple feels a loss of control. They might have planned the birth with great care, then suddenly their world is turned upside down and they realize how little control they have over many of life's important events. As with other cases of perceived loss of control, depression can follow if the parents are not able to cope with their feelings.

Probably the nicest part of having unexpected twins is that they are unexpected. Parents who know that they are expecting twins worry over potential difficulties that can arise both with the mother and the twins. If twins are unexpected, parents are calmer. However, prepared for only one birth, parents often do not have the resources to buy sufficient diapers and clothes, or to place the twins away from each other while they are sleeping. They might need financial relief and will certainly need about ten additional hours each day to make up for the sleep that they will miss during the nights to come.

Early in their stay at the hospital, the parents will need to adjust their conception of their family size and composition. After living for seven or so months with the idea that they would be a family of three, adjusting to being a family of four requires some getting used to. Most of the other problems of adjustment are similar to parents in which the twins were expected prior to birth.

Advance Preparation for Multiple Births

About one of every eight or so births in the United States is a multiple birth.[1] Many women are happy with giving birth to twins because they get two babies by going through only one pregnancy, labor and delivery. To many, that seems quite a bargain.

However, the health risks to both mother and babies are greater. Mothers of multiple babies are more likely to develop anemia, polyhydramnios (excess amniotic fluid in the uterus), hemorrhage before birth, some types of diabetes, and toxemia (involving high blood pressure, retention of protein in the urine, and swelling due to fluid retention, which can be fatal).[2]

The risks to the preborn twins are even worse.[3] The chance for miscarriage is higher in women pregnant with multiple than with single babies, as is the chance of stillbirth for one or both babies. Twins or other multiples are more likely to be aborted than are singletons. Finally, the youngest twin is more likely to die shortly after birth than single babies or than the first-born twin. Thus, the risk of infant mortality with pregnancies involving multiple babies is greater than with single babies. If the twins survive, they are more likely than singletons to be premature, of low birth weight, to present themselves for delivery in difficult positions, and to have some congenital birth defects (such as club foot, excess fingers or toes, anomalies, and spina bifida—in order of decreasing likelihood).

The risks of infant death, deformity, or other difficulty are not the only issues facing the parents of twins. They are likely also to be called upon to make important decisions during the pregnancy. They might have to decide whether to allow x-rays or whether to permit an amniocentesis, or how to deal with the discovery of a deformed child.

Several other aspects of having a pregnancy with multiples involve rapid early weight-gain. Even during the first three months of pregnancy, the mother will usually begin to show. Her weight-gain for the birth of twins will be perhaps half again as much as with the birth of a singleton. One danger of the late discovery of a multiple pregnancy is that the mother has been trying to maintain her body weight at a level that would be correct for a single pregnancy.

When news is not perceived as "good news," such as when a couple discovers that a multiple birth will place enormous financial burdens on them or when they discover that the child is deformed, there is a tendency to deny the reality of the news. It is especially important that they plan specifically how they intend to cope with the birth of the children. They might read books about having twins.[4] They might also visit ongoing support groups for parents of twins or couples who are currently parenting twins to discuss the likely problems they will encounter.

Coping with two newborns will be challenging—to say the least—so it is helpful if the parents arrange for necessary support services before the birth. Because of the increased likelihood that the twins will be premature, it is generally helpful to make arrangements at the beginning of the third trimester of pregnancy. Help might be obtained from the parents' parents or from church or neighborhood friends. In other cases, the couple might hire someone to help with the children or with household duties for as long as a year after the birth of the children. In cases where funds are limited, the couple might enlist the help of a responsible high school student or of a senior citizen to assist the mother. The father might also arrange vacation time or flexible work hours to make the adjustment to twins easier.

After the birth, the woman will usually need to do postpartum physical exercises to help get her body back into physical shape necessary to handle the twins.

PREPARING FOR BACK-TO-BACK PREGNANCIES

Imagine this. You are tired. The parent, especially the mother, of an infant less than one year old is always tired. During the course of the day, you have changed about twenty diapers, run two miles trying to see why the child is crying, fed the child his or her one solid food (strained peas), done two loads of laundry, washed dishes, swept, dusted, read half a book entitled *Helping Your Infant Learn,* experienced every emotion known to the human species, missed a meal, and noticed a new varicose vein in your leg. At night you stay awake until after ten nursing the baby, then gratefully fall into sweet sleep. Until one o'clock, when it is again time to feed the child. At three o'clock you awaken to the cry of the child, whereupon you discern that it sounds like a wet diaper cry. The husband is awakened to tend to the baby. At six o'clock you awaken to the sound of the alarm and the cheerful gurgling of the baby. Eagerly you swing your legs out of bed, take a deep breath, smile, and run, suddenly queasy, for the bathroom threatening with a rude greeting anyone in your path. Congratulations: You are morning sick. Again.

You suddenly realize that the tiredness you have felt since the beginning of the last pregnancy is not going to get better soon. In fact, the prospect of being tired all through the morning sickness of the first trimester of pregnancy and through the heaviness of the last trimester of pregnancy—or, to phrase it differently, to be sick and heavy throughout the first year of your child's life—are not pleasant prospects. You had kind of looked forward to experiencing tiredness as a pure experience. Now the pregnancy has cut that short.

The Challenge to Mothering Skills

The infant requires almost constant attention. The mother feels "on duty" sixteen hours a day and "on call" for the other eight hours. To help the young child develop, it is necessary to maintain one's equanimity. The mother who is depressed or frustrated will often be more upset with her baby's behavior than the mother who is not depressed or frustrated. This theory, which is supported by empirical research, is called the "threshold theory."[5] It hypothesizes that when the mother is emotionally upset, she has a lower threshold for troublesome behavior than when she is not upset; she will thus define the behavior as needing professional attention more easily than when she is not emotionally upset. Although research has not addressed the question directly, this threshold theory suggests that the mother who is pregnant might be more likely to define her infant's behavior as troublesome than if she were not pregnant. The addition of the pregnancy to the normal trials of child rearing thus presents strong challenges to the mother.

The Challenge to Marriage

Raising an infant who is less than one year of age is a challenge. The parent is generally reeling from the marital interruptions that accompany the birth of a child. The couple's time schedules were likely disrupted and thus their patterns of intimacy were altered; the new parents probably feel they are "never" alone with each other. As they try to regain stable patterns of behaving in which they can meet their need for intimacy, coaction, and distance, the new pregnancy is discovered. Their time schedules are about to be affected again, while they are still somewhat unstable from the previous disruption.

New opportunities present themselves for decisions. What will this child be named? Where will the baby sleep? How will we prevent the two children from keeping each other awake all night? Should we go through Lamaze classes again? Will we have this child by using the Lamaze method? Any issues that were not firmly resolved (and some that were) will have to be renegotiated once again while the memory of the discussions are still fresh imprints on the mind.

COPING WITH TWINS

Dealing with pregnancies in the event of multiple births or when children are closely spaced is not the end of the challenge. It is just the beginning. Once the birth(s) occur, adjustment is needed in raising twins or closely spaced siblings.

The First Days

Coping with twins begins even before leaving the hospital. Often the physician will offer some sage advice, "I'd recommend that you cancel all appointments for a while—about two years."

What makes the first few days difficult is the combination of factors. First, there is tiredness from the labor and delivery. Then, there is the grueling experience of staying in the hospital and fitting into hospital routine. Sitz baths are nice, but being awakened in order to take a sleeping pill and then not being able to return to sleep gets old. Third, the hormones are wildly gyrating as the milk comes in and the body seeks to stabilize itself. Once the mother goes home the demands of caring for the infants are staggering—even if she has help with the housework from relatives, father, friends, or neighbors. Merely feeding twins is a full-time job, not to mention changing diapers, giving baths, and changing their clothes. Feelings of being overwhelmed can be difficult to handle soon after the birth. The woman anticipates the time when she will be left to care for the infants alone, and the result is a feeling of helplessness and powerlessness. During this time, she needs considerable support and assurance from friends and from her husband.

After Grandmother Goes Home

After the adjustment period, the parents assume the child-rearing duties without much outside assistance. Most parents of twins feel restricted, much more so than with the birth of a single child. Babysitters are often hard to find or expensive. The typical high-school sophomore feels inadequate for the task of handling infant twins. Being asked about babysitting for two infants, the high-school sophomore usually exercises creative excuse-making capabilities. "I think I'm going to have a date that night. If not, I might be sick." Many couples learn to bring their entertainment home to them by fixing special meals together, renting videotape players and several movies over a weekend, or simply packing up the children in strollers and/or backpacks and walking around the neighborhood.

Twins break down social barriers, as the parents soon find

out. Neighbors stroll to meet the couple on the street. "Oh, aren't they cute. Whew, I'm glad it's you and not us. I don't know how we would cope with two at the same time."

Comments like that warm the heart and inspire confidence in the parents of new twins. After a while, though, the parents learn to accept the public attention. Fathers often say that despite the extra work that twins entail, they feel that the public attention they receive makes it more than worth it.

The children, too, benefit from increased attention. Perhaps twins receive somewhat less attention from their parents than single babies might, but this is generally more than compensated for by the increased attention that twins receive from others—including complete strangers. Parents of twins quickly become accustomed to strangers patting and talking to the twins.

Handling Daily Demands of Raising Twins

The parents must learn to handle the quantity and variety of demands they will face as parents of twins. For example, a crying infant can test the patience of most parents, but twins often sing duets. Parents must learn to handle the frustration of two crying babies when there is no apparent reason for their crying.

Sleeping is often a problem. Usually, it is helpful to try to get the twins adjusted to the same sleeping schedule. But twins are sometimes not amenable to that parental suggestion. When one twin is considerably larger than the other, the larger twin will often require less sleep. When one twin awakens, he or she often awakens the other. Parents of twins often remove the phone from the hook during their infants' nap time. That is the only time that the mother can catch a nap to compensate for the missed sleep during the night. In many households of twins, the babies must sleep in the same room, or even the same bed. If the twins' needs for sleep are approximately the same, this proximity helps place the twins on the same schedule.

Housework multiplies. Each family must find a way to cope with routine housework while meeting the child-care demands of the twins. For some families, this will require hiring a student, elderly person, or professional to help. For other families, the husband will assume more of the household maintenance duties. One mother of twins told me that her solution was to get up a half-hour earlier than everyone else. This gave her thirty uninterrupted minutes at the beginning of each day to get the house in order. She said that the family simply learned to sleep through her housecleaning routine. Others have fixed lunches en masse—sandwiches for the week are prepared while watching television one night. One woman fixed lunch during breakfast time each morning, refrigerating the sandwiches until lunch time.

Raising Two Individuals

Parents of twins want each twin to be treated as a unique individual. Little effort should be spent correcting and educating others about calling each twin by name rather than referring to them jointly as "the twins." Rather, the family will be the base of support for the twins, and family members can establish separateness by simply treating the twins as individuals.

Calling each twin by name—and not making a mistake—is difficult. We don't have twins and I find myself calling roll in order to get one child's attention. I don't know why the average parent cannot remember the name of his or her children in the midst of a command, but virtually every parent does this. With twins, it is especially important that parents try to keep their names straight. If parents make mistakes, their children will usually let them know, though children are unlikely to correct teachers and other adults.

It is also important that parents not compare one twin with the other. Comparison stimulates competition and can induce twins to compete strongly with each other, or one may avoid doing things that the sibling enjoys so competition can be avoided. This competition can extend into adulthood.[6]

Building separate identities in twins requires being sensitive to their individual needs. As twins, the babies will often have similar needs, even as they grow older. The parents must not force separateness on them. For example, some parents of twins have required them to choose separate activities or sports so that they would be assured of different experiences.

Because the twins might have similar interests, this artificial choice among activities might deny them the opportunity to excel at something at which they were gifted. On the other hand, the parent must help the twins gain independence. This is best promoted through helping children develop their individual skills and praising them for their performance. Usually, we recommend that each twin be praised alone rather than in front of his or her sibling, for that can stimulate competition.

One skill that is important to develop is language. Twins are usually later to develop language than single babies. The most frequent speech model for a twin is the other twin—who also doesn't talk. Sometimes twins even create a private language, called twin-speech or cryptophasia. It is important for the parents to talk frequently to the twins from birth. Even though the twins cannot understand the parent, the parent allows the twins to hear the rhythm of language. This also trains the parent to talk to the twins, which will facilitate the twins' learning language when they become old enough to learn.

COPING WITH TWO CLOSE-TOGETHER CHILDREN

Kirby and I have four children, each spaced two years apart. We think that spacing is ideal, though some people cringe and say they need more time to recover between children. We have not had to deal with two children less than a year apart. To me that seems extreme. Few parents plan it that way; it just happens.

Twins go in two different directions at the same time. Two infants separated by a year or less go in two different directions at the same time, but at different rates. They also team up to wreck things around the house systematically, but that usually comes later—in their second year.

If the births are timed right, the fortunate parent can even learn to deal with two two-year-olds simultaneously. The incidence of the word "no" in that household would stagger the imagination. For instance, the older two-year-old runs to the coffee table and places her chair on top of it. When the mother sees that, she says, "No, no, dear. Chairs belong on the floor. Take it down."

"No."

"No, no, dear. Don't say no to Mommy."

The younger two-year-old totters into the living room at that very instant with the end of the toilet paper in her hand.

"No!" the mother says, aghast.

"No?" responds the toddler.

"No," says Mom. She begins to trace the trail of toilet paper through every room of the house. As she enters the bathroom with an armful of toilet paper, "Noooo." She has just discovered the diaper pail has been overturned on the rug.

The two-year-olds look at each other. "Nooo," they imitate. They are working on developing patience in their mother. It is usually better not to forewarn mothers of close-together children about these developmental experiences.

Coping with Two Children Under One Year Old

What is it like to raise two infants separated by less than one year of age?

I walked slowly toward the door of the red brick, ranch-style house. Two trees graced the front yard and tulips were in bloom in front of the soon-to-flower azalea bushes along the front of the house. An air of innocence graced the house and yard. Pushing the lighted bell, I heard the wail of a police car in the distance, soon joined by another. Mrs. Howe answered the door, a nine-month infant balanced on her hip.

"Come in, Dr. Worthington. I've been expecting you."

"Thank you for allowing me to interview you, Mrs. Howe."

She motioned toward a chair. "Roddy, the young one, is asleep, now, but he is due to get up any minute. And Tom is all rested up. He had a nap earlier this afternoon, before Roddy went down. I almost timed it right. You said you wanted to see what it was like when both the boys were awake."

Mrs. Howe had agreed to be interviewed about how she coped with two young children. She and her husband had tried to conceive for five years without success. They had spent three years on a waiting list for adoption before adopting Tom, and then, just after the adoption was approved, they discovered that she was pregnant. Now the Howes were coping with a nine-month-old and two-month-old.

After a few moments of conversation, Roddy signaled, loudly, that he was awake and ready to be entertained. I had forgotten how loudly a two-month-old could signal. Mrs. Howe placed Tom on the carpet and zipped off toward the bedroom. As she disappeared, Tom popped up to his knees and crawled directly to the coffee table. Reaching up, he hoisted himself to a standing position on what seemed like shaky legs. He looked around, oblivious to me, and reached over toward a pile of *Popular Mechanics* magazines stacked on the coffee table. *Now there's a precocious kid*, I thought to myself, whereupon he lost his balance as the magazines slipped and he pirouetted to the floor via the edge of the coffee table.

Immediately, he signaled his anguish. I noticed his signal system was much better developed than even younger brother Roddy's. In ran his mother with a half-diapered, screaming two-month-old glued to her hip. She looked accusingly at me.

"He fell," I said helplessly, thinking she might have suspected me of child abuse. Laying Roddy on the couch, she saw his unpinned diaper fall away as she picked up Tom. That's when I heard a sound that was out of place in the living room: running water.

"Roddy, *no*," yelled Mrs. Howe, which startled Roddy, who spread the damage over more of the living room carpet, and (I confess) drenched my shoe, too.

Both children were still crying. Louder than ever. Mrs. Howe glanced frantically at me and I could read in her eyes the haunted look of the pursued animal. With one hand, she covered Roddy. She apologized to me and soothed both children in the same sentence.

"Can I help?" I asked.

"No," she said. "It'll calm down in a minute." Tom, the older, was already beginning to survey the potted plants thoughtfully. I guessed that, if things ran true to form, he would probably eat them. No such luck. The unmistakable sound of his messy bowel movement echoed through the room. It got everyone's attention.

"Incredible timing," Mrs. Howe said. We looked at each other. "Maybe you can help. Would you mind diapering little Roddy, while I change Tom?"

171

"Not at all," I said. "I have four of my own and this keeps the old skills sharp."

"Good." She rushed into the bedroom and emerged quickly with a dry cloth diaper for little Roddy. Then she disappeared again to perform the dirty work. I noticed a path worn in the carpet between couch and bedroom.

"Let's be friends," I offered in what I thought was a conciliatory gesture toward the still wailing Roddy. Just then he smacked me on the nose. I suspected he had been secretly watching Hulk Hogan on television when he was supposed to be taking naps. He wanted to wrestle. I outweighed him by about 150 pounds, though. With only a little difficulty, I wrestled him onto a towel on the floor and pinned him—that is, I subdued him without literally pinning him. He still protested loudly to the referee, but I completed the diaper lock with what I thought to be great poise. The rubber pants were nowhere to be found, apparently forgotten in Mrs. Howe's rush to help Randy when he had fallen. So I picked up little Roddy and began to bounce him, thinking that at least he probably wouldn't burp on me because he had just awakened from his nap and had not yet eaten. He entertained himself for thirty long seconds by intertwining the fingers of both hands in my beard and swinging back and forth. This increased the blood flow to my cheeks—which will probably speed the healing.

Mrs. Howe returned with a clean, dry, and happy Tom just as I became aware that my shirt felt wet. "Roddy, you rascal," I said with a somewhat forced smile. "I thought you had finished with that when you got my shoe." The coward was afraid to answer, but I thought I detected a malicious smile even among his continuing tears.

His mother, taking little Roddy from me and placing Tom on the floor, disappeared again to wherever she kept the clean diapers. Let's see, that seemed like about six sets of diapers in the twenty minutes I had been here. At that rate, I calculated she would have to wash about two hundred per day. Fourteen hundred per week. Five thousand six hundred per month. I broke into an empathic sweat, drenching the back of my shirt.

Happily, Tom crawled over to me and chinned himself on the knee that was dry, raising a friction burn, and pulling out

172

most of the hair on my thigh. I smiled and lifted him to my lap, where he burped on my pants. "Mrs. Howe," I said, "I take it that Tom and Roddy are not on the same feeding schedules."

"Heavens, no," she shouted back from the bedroom. "That would be far too easy. I just finished feeding Tom before you came."

Thirty minutes later I walked out of the innocent-looking house and headed to my car, a broken man in a broken suit. Mrs. Howe apologized to me because we had had so little time to talk about what it was like to have two children under the age of one year old. Funny, I think I had an inkling.

Effects on the Marriage

Like any birth, close-together births both disrupt the parents' time schedules and provide opportunities for the couple to reconsider decisions that they thought had just been resolved. The potential is thus present for the marriage to be weakened or strengthened. Having concentrated on the potential for weakening the marriage when I discussed the pregnancy, I will now mention some ways that the marriage might be strengthened by a second birth.

Intimacy might be strengthened for a couple of reasons. Because child-care responsibilities will be increased, a husband and wife will have the opportunity to divide household chores and do some of the tasks together that were previously done by one spouse alone.

Furthermore, most people in the couple's social circle will know that they now have two infants to care for. Generally, they will understand the extra effort required and will thus provide social approval when the father asks for extra time for the family. As a caveat, the spouses must be sure to make time for each other. The demands for child care can consume all the "family time." The couple must continue to plan activities that they can enjoy together—both with and without the children.

Because the husband and wife have usually been forced to make a number of child rearing decisions within the past year, those decisions are fresh in their minds. They can use the new decisions to reinforce and strengthen their earlier decisions, thus adding additional stability to the family. Generally, this can be accomplished if they are not engaged in ongoing power struggles.

COUNSELING THE COUPLE WITH TWINS OR CLOSE BIRTHS

Under *most* circumstances, a couple with a strong marriage will be able to deal with most stresses and strains of multiple or close births *if* they have the information, skills, and social support necessary, and *if* they are not overwhelmed by other stressful life events occurring simultaneously. When couples seek counseling for their difficulties, I usually make the following assessments:

1. How strong is the marriage?

2. How have the couple's time schedules been disrupted by the multiple or close births and what effect has the disruption had on their intimacy?

3. How many unresolved issues must be decided?

4. How much is the conflict a product of the situation and how much is it a long-standing power struggle for which the births merely provide opportunities to exert their positions?

5. Do they have accurate and sufficient information about the event they are facing?

6. Do they have the relationship skills to hold their marriage at a high functioning level? Do they have the parenting skills to accomplish the tasks required of them?

7. Do they have social support from relatives, church friends, other friends, and co-workers that empower them to work together to solve their problems, or are social support systems aligned to support spouses against each other?

8. What other life events are they dealing with simultaneously?

Based on the answers to these questions, I will design a treatment for the couple, maximizing their involvement in solving their difficulties and minimizing my role as counselor. The marriage will be strengthened to the extent that the man and woman can pull together, relying on themselves and on the work of God in their lives to solve their problem.

I view the counselor as a consultant who will help the couple gather the resources—information, skills, social support—they need to create more stable time schedules, more intimacy, better decisions with less conflict, and an end to power struggles. I might do that through referring the couple to readings, tapes, support groups (such as the Mothers of Twins clubs), or training groups (such as parenting skills groups). Or I might help the couple improve their marriage as a precursor to working on their problems with their children. Or, in the event of an already strong marriage, I might coach the couple about how to deal with their children at various ages. Finally, if other transitions impinge on their adjustment, I will help them deal with the other transitions as well as with their children.

Although as a human I enjoy being appreciated and respected for the help I can provide, I know that the couple will experience more lasting change if they place their trust in the Lord rather than in the counsel of humans. This does not negate any counsel or advice that I might give. People are the body of Christ, and we are his hands, his mouthpiece, his feet. He can and often does intervene in people's lives sovereignly, but he works through his body, too.

PREVENTION

Few people intentionally try to have children within a year of each other. Fewer still set their sights on twins. Prevention of the problems with multiple or close births can only be secondary prevention. Intervention can occur with couples who already know they are going to have twins or who are pregnant with a due date that falls within a year or so of an earlier child. Usually the intervention will involve sharing books and other information. Most couples do not reach the "teachable moment" until the birth is closer—within the last trimester of pregnancy or immediately after birth. Thus, as a counselor, my best strategy is to educate myself about the trials and stresses of twins and close births and to maintain a reading list and a small collection of books that deal with the problem. Then I will be prepared when the difficulty arises.

PART THREE

PREGNANCIES THAT ARE TOO LATE OR NEVER

CHAPTER EIGHT

THY QUIVER OVERFLOWETH: ONE CHILD TOO MANY AND CHILDREN WITH SPECIAL PROBLEMS

Lo, sons are a heritage from the Lord, the fruit of the womb a reward. Like arrows in the hand of a warrior are the sons of one's youth. Happy is the man who has his quiver full of them! (Ps. 127:3–5)

SOMETIMES THE QUIVER IS FULL and the automatic arrowmaker is stuck in the open position. Thy quiver is scheduled to overflow in the next nine months. It's no joking matter. It makes you quiver just to think about it.

WHEN CAN A CHILD BE ONE TOO MANY?

There are several times when the quiver can overflow with what at first seems like too much of a good thing. One instance might be when the problem is created by multiple births. Some parents might be so excited by multiple births that they can hardly believe their census. On the other hand, suppose a couple had planned to have two children. In their second pregnancy, they become the proud parents of quintuplets—or even twins. Besides dealing with the difficulties of a multiple birth (see chapter 7), this father and mother will have to adjust their lives to manage one too many—one more than they had thought possible.

A second instance in which a baby might be thought of as "one too many" is when a couple has decided that their family is complete—but God has decided it is not. In the old joke, the baby is born with an apparently deformed hand, but upon closer examination, it is tightly clutching a birth control pill. That baby will take some getting used to. It is the "whoops-baby."

A third instance of the seemingly "one too many" baby occurs when the couple intentionally gets pregnant with a baby that is wanted and prayed for. But after its birth, the family finds out that they have exceeded their quiver size. This is like the Peter Principle in business in which executives are continually promoted until they reach a level at which they cannot perform effectively. In the Parents' Peter Principle, the parents continue to have children until they find they have had one too many.

A fourth instance involves changes in the status of the family after the pregnancy. Perhaps the husband loses his job. Or the stock market fails. For whatever reason, the family finds that "things have changed" since the child was conceived.

A child might also appear to be "one too many" because the child requires more work, attention, or just sacrificial love than had been anticipated. This might be true of the child who is merely a difficult baby—fussing, crying, restless at every opportunity. It might be because the child is deformed, or retarded, or chronically ill. In each of those instances, the family fabric will be strained and stretched. All of these cases will be discussed in this chapter.

A final instance of the quiver overflowing might involve a menopause baby or one conceived during mid-life. A couple has spent twenty years raising a family. Just as the last child prepares to leave home, the parents discover that a "new" last child is about to be born. Counseling the mid-life family with a new baby is discussed in chapter 9.

As I have listed the reasons that a child might be perceived to be "one too many," I have carefully said "appeared to be" or "perceived to be" one too many. I believe, of course, that God knows what is best for us and that he often gives us what *we* think are too many trials when they are actually just enough to accomplish God's purposes.

On the other hand, I also believe that humans make responsible choices that have real consequences. One of those consequences might be the birth of a child that God did not originally have in mind as his perfect will for us. However, once we have made the choice, God wants us to move beyond the belief that the child is "one too many," unplanned, unloved. He wants us to value the human life he has entrusted to us and care for it as if it were part of our own body. Given my assumptions, it should not be surprising that one of my aims in counseling couples discussed in this chapter is to help them accept the child as a valuable member of their family.

"ONE TOO MANY"

Having "one too many" is not a condition. It is a perception, a judgment. The parents think their family is complete, but then they discover they are pregnant, or their financial circumstances or living arrangements change. Or, the judgment may be made after the child's birth, such as when parents feel overwhelmed by the multitude of child-care and child-rearing tasks.

Why do people develop the perception that this particular child is "one too many"? Perceived costs outweigh benefits. Perceived costs and benefits include both immediate and delayed costs and benefits. Delayed costs and benefits both appear to be worth less in the present moment than they will when the future finally arrives.

With this understanding, it is possible to help the family change perceived costs and benefits of the new child. Either the family members can change the *actual* costs and benefits, or the family members can work directly to change the perceptions. Changing actual costs and benefits will usually result in changes in the way family members perceive the cost-benefit balance, but in some cases the change in perception does not occur. Generally, that might be the case when the family member *discounts* or devalues the change.

Jim, for example, believes that *if only* he can find a second job, the extra income would relieve the financial pressure and he and Sally would no longer resent their infant son. When he finally finds a second job, he discovers that there are many other things that he has resented. And now he resents having to put out the extra effort to hold a second job. He has devalued the solution until it is no solution at all.

Increasing Actual Benefits of Having a Child

Of all the ways to solve the apparent problem of one too many children, increasing the actual benefits of having the child is the most difficult. Having a child *is* a benefit from God (Ps. 127:3). Perhaps the easiest way to increase the benefits is to increase family intimacy. Older siblings can be involved as much as possible in some of the child care—even if they "help" by watching. Parents can work together on some of the child-care duties, increasing the time they spend together. The couple can spend time together also in planning ways to handle the increased duties around the house.

After the birth of our fourth child, Kirby and I spent many nights walking around the block and talking about ways that we could rearrange family duties to make everyone happier. I now look back on this time as a blessing, though for a time we had some disruption in our normal schedules.

Decreasing Actual Costs of Having a Child

Economic costs. Economic costs can be defrayed by either increasing family income or by decreasing family expenditures. In the last fifteen years, people in the United States have emphasized increasing income. Many women have felt the "necessity" to return to the work force even though they did not enjoy the work. What most have found is that the wages brought in by a second wage earner are often largely used up by extra child-care costs, extra wardrobe costs, purchase of additional convenience foods, eating out more frequently, additional automotive expenses, and paying more income tax. The standard of living is increased and what once were luxuries become necessities. Furthermore, the entire lifestyle of the family is transformed when there are two wage earners rather than one.

A second way to defray the economic costs of the child is to spend less money. At our church, many of the couples are in their childbearing years. They pass baby clothes around the congregation. Each Sunday after church, the trip to the car is like Christmas. How many bags of clothes will we find in the car this week? And for whom? One week a friend jokingly said, "We really made out this week. We dropped off three bags of clothes and only were given two bags."

Another way to defray costs is to frequent yard sales. In our end of town, there are usually twenty yard sales each Saturday. The newspaper has an entire column or more that advertises yard sales. Many people do not even advertise in the paper. Generally, we take care of many of our children's Christmas presents and household needs through yard sales. But beware the yard sale addict. One man always arrives in a cloud of dust with a stare that is strangely focused on the distant horizon. Sweeping through the articles, he spots an item he needs. Stomping large items and small children, he beats his way to the item, casually hoists it and begins to dicker with the owner over price. This man is probably a floor broker on the New York Stock Exchange during the week. He brings the same intensity to yard-sale bargaining sessions. The unsuspecting owner can walk away from the "bargain" receiving two dollars and thirty-seven cents for a riding lawn mower in mint condition if not careful. Despite the hazards, yard sales are excellent ways to reduce expenditures.

Grocery costs can also be reduced through buying marked-down food, day-old bread, dented cans, and by using coupons. Comparative shopping seems to be a dying art, but it is possible to save hundreds of dollars each year by smart grocery shopping.

What often worries parents is not just the immediate expenses. Parents worry about how their child will be put through college or started in business or given a large wedding. Generally, these future expenses can be taken care of through either saving or securing loans when the expenses are due. For many people, saving money is difficult, though it provides the most direct answer to financial worries. Most employers have programs that allow employees to save a portion of their income for retirement or other personal reasons.

Finally, economic costs can be reduced through careful budgeting, which lessens impulsive buying. A number of books about the financial management of household funds are on the market, so I will not discuss this further. The couple feeling the financial strain can be referred to one of those books for help. In addition, usually someone within most congregations is able to give sound financial advice and counsel to couples who wish to manage their finances more efficiently.

Effort. The effort of childrearing can often be reduced through doing tasks more efficiently. Kathy White's "Motherhood as a Career" group at our church has provided a forum for mothers to exchange ideas about how to do the task of motherhood. Other ways that effort can be reduced might include hiring work done or encouraging volunteering within the church community to help the overwhelmed family.

Personal support. Burdens seem lighter when they are shared. Overwhelmed parents can share their burdens by maintaining a support network, which might include a regular weekly or monthly group meeting. Usually the group meeting will be supplemented by a telephone network. Individual meetings and visits with friends allow time for more personal sharing.

Cost to the marriage. The cost of an unplanned pregnancy to the marriage involves disrupted time schedules, decreased intimacy, and the effort of learning new roles. Making changes in the marriage relationship requires thoughtful planning, determined action, and self-control. The couple must decide that they value their relationship enough to improve it. By planning specific changes that they intend to make, they provide a goal and the motivation to work toward it.

Resources for parenthood. Parenthood requires effort to locate resources to help with handling difficulties. A church can provide a valuable service to couples by collecting and maintaining a resource file on the difficulties of parenthood and how to cope with them. To create such a resource file, you as counselor may suggest that a class be formed—either a Sunday school or midweek class on Christian parenting. You may be the one to conduct the class, or one of the older parents in the church. Those who attend should be encouraged to share their resources: lists of good books, tapes, pamphlets, or other helpful material. The class might be encouraged to donate their favorite resources to the church so that other families might have easy access to the materials. A master file, organized under topic, can be created by someone in the class with organizational skill so that the list and resources can be continually expanded and can be easily used by others.

Changing Perceptions of the Costs and Benefits of Having a Child

Changing one's thoughts is not easy. Most people have tried to change their thoughts on numerous occasions, but on only few of those occasions do their thoughts actually change. Why? Usually they are not trying to change their thoughts efficiently. Some common strategies people use are downright counterproductive. There are three common mistakes people make in trying to change their thoughts, and I warn against these in counseling.

1. Don't say *don't*. When people realize they are thinking about their child as being "one too many" or as being a burden, they generally admonish themselves *not* to think that way. *Don't think about how much extra work this child causes. Don't think about how resentful you feel. And don't think about the deprivation of the other children because all of your energy is going toward caring for this infant.*

This is about as effective as instructing oneself not to think about oranges, about how the juice spurts from them when they are cut, about how the tangy taste tingles on the sides of the tongue. Obviously, as you read these words, you thought about oranges. Instructing oneself "don't think about . . ." merely calls the image to mind. The mind ignores the word *don't* and goes directly to the image. When I demonstrate this to a church-based seminar, I tell the people not to think of oranges as I describe in detail how not to think about them.

"Did you think about oranges?" I ask.

Heads bob. Inevitably, one hand goes up. "I didn't," says the person smugly. The smugness is mixed with a half-defensive posture as if the person expected me to jump the four rows of seats and throttle his or her neck.

"How did you do it?" I asked, puzzled.

"I thought about apples."

"Great," I usually answer. "That demonstrates a great spiritual principle. We cannot solve our problems by focusing on the problems. We only make ourselves more miserable by doing that. We can only solve our problems by focusing on the solution. Jesus is the solution. *He* can reveal through faith and for faith how we can solve problems. Jesus must be the apple of our eye."

2. Don't repeat yourself. We often think we can brainwash ourselves into changing our thoughts by constantly repeating good thoughts. This rarely works. These are "vain repetitions" and Jesus cautioned the Pharisees against them. Saying the same positive sentences repetitively soon erodes the meaning from the sentences, leaving a meaningless mantra. The Hindus and Buddhists use repetitive mantras to empty the mind of content. An empty mind is only a temporary solution to problems. Stay away from senseless repetitions.

3. Don't hit and run. People must *systematically* change their thoughts. One reason that people fail to change their thoughts is that they try it for about thirty minutes and then give up. Changing any habit requires extended and systematic practice. The same is true with changing one's perceptions.

Thus, three guidelines for changing perceptions can be derived from reversing the common mistakes people make: focus on Jesus and seek his direction for solutions, concentrate on thinking out solutions rather than on repetitions, and systematically and continually try to change negative thinking.

Three other guidelines are helpful, I tell those whom I counsel. First, compartmentalize difficulties. When we become overwhelmed, we often allow the distress and depression to pervade our lives. Rather, learn to place problems into compartments. Enjoy the positive times in family life without allowing the worries to intrude. Often this can be accomplished by setting aside a "worry time" in the evening when problems can be thought about. During the remainder of the day, simply remind yourself that there will be time to think about that later, then move on to more positive thinking.

Second, whatever one thinks about dominates the emotional state. Simply focusing on distractions from the problems can help change perceptions.

Third, reframe problems. Problems can be seen in other lights. Usually, it is difficult to reframe the problems as "strengths" or "opportunities" because we are so involved in them. However, pretend that you have been given a creativity test. Try to think of how many positive aspects there are to the situation that formerly seemed so dismal and overwhelming.

The key to changing perceptions is that whatever people think about will act as a filter through which events and circumstances pass. If our thoughts are focused on God, we will see solutions that he has for us. If our thoughts are focused on our difficulties, we will only see additional difficulties.

COUNSELING FAMILIES WHO THINK THEY HAVE "ONE TOO MANY"

Although the problem of "one too many" is a perceptual problem, the counselor cannot expect to merely outline the logical alternatives and see the problem disappear. From the perspective of the family, the problem is emotional rather than logical. The counselor must establish emotional connectedness with the mother and father before they will be open to logical solutions to their difficulties.

The counselor must allow the family to express the difficulties they are having with the new child or the difficulties they expect to have when the child is born. Only when difficulties have been enumerated should the counselor gently focus the attention of the couple or family on possible solutions. Emotion is a product of physiological arousal and appraisal of the situation. The counselor must attempt to reduce the emotion by lowering both components of the emotion.

Arousal is lowered through providing hope for the family.

The counselor might share accounts of other desperate families and describe how their family relationships turned around. The counselor might reassure the family, though generally glib reassurances will be ineffective. The counselor can build hope through having family members recall other difficult times in their lives and remember how the Lord worked with them to bring them through that crisis. Finally, the family can be told to think through the Bible and find examples of how God was faithful with his people, even when they thought life was the darkest.

The appraisal of the situation is affected by involving family members in some of the thinking I have outlined above. They can be helped to change their actual benefits and costs with the child and to perceive the situation differently. Because the focus of attention of family members is crucial to success, the counselor must involve the family in tasks that have them challenge their negative perceptions and exert energy in developing more positive perceptions.

DIFFICULT CHILDREN

About 10 percent of all babies might be called "difficult babies."[1] They cry almost incessantly, sleep fitfully, and seem impossible to please. Parents of difficult babies generally experience great stress. They miss sleep, which lowers their threshold to discomfort. They also experience the full range of emotions. They generally are frustrated because they cannot calm the baby. Frustration changes to anger. Parents of difficult babies often report the urge to harm the child and research has shown that some parents follow through on these urges at times. Difficult babies have a higher risk of maltreatment than normal babies.[2] Anger can easily change to depression when parents, weakened by loss of sleep, begin to feel they are powerless to please or calm the baby. Guilt can be present even if parents do not mistreat the child. Violent thoughts suggest to parents that something must be wrong with them. They often feel as if they are not fit parents because they cannot please the baby. Social withdrawal might occur along with loss of self-confidence and lowered self-esteem.

As a secondary consequence, parents might neglect the baby because being a parent is not as rewarding as they had desired it to be. The result is a vicious circle in which both parents and child do not experience pleasant and happy development. Even older children are affected by the difficult baby. Six-year-old Marie asked her mother about the new baby, Nick. "Honey," replied her mother, "Nick is a real gift from heaven."

Marie replied: "I guess God must have wanted it quieter up there, huh?"

Counseling parents of difficult babies requires providing information, skills, and support. Knowing the high incidence of difficult children can often relieve parents' guilt. In addition, knowing that it is not uncommon to entertain fantasies of harming the child can help parents handle the feelings. The counselor needs to encourage parents to develop ways to handle an infant's crying rather than resorting to abuse or neglect.

Some skills can be developed for handling prolonged crying by the difficult infant. Parents can learn to "tune out" the crying and to "tune in" other thoughts. Parents can recognize the stages of their building frustration and anger or depression and ward off negative feelings at early stages instead of letting them build until they are uncontrollable. Parents can learn to take "time out" from the baby in order to plan how they will cope with the crying during their attempts to settle the infant down. Other skills for handling difficult infants have been described in work by Kirkland, who established a call-in clinic for parents of difficult infants—CrySOS[3] (see Appendix 4 for some recommended readings).

MENTALLY RETARDED CHILDREN

Mental retardation refers to mental impairment sufficient to prevent a child from functioning effectively in comparison to his or her age mates.[4] The causes of mental retardation might include inheritance, injury during or after birth, chemical abnormalities during pregnancy, environmental impoverishment, or any of a number of causes. There are over two hundred identified causes of mental retardation.[5]

Degree of mental retardation usually is measured in terms of intelligence quotient (IQ). An IQ of 100 would indicate a child who is average relative to his or her peers. A large majority of the population (95 percent) falls between an IQ of about 70 and 130, depending on the test used to measure the IQ. Children who have IQs from 50 to 70 are usually called mildly retarded. Most develop skills equivalent to fifth-grade children and many are self-supporting as adults.

Children with IQs between 25 and 50 are described as moderately mentally retarded. They generally will ultimately handle some social relationships and can learn to care for themselves. Children with IQs lower than 25 are called profoundly mentally retarded and most are generally totally dependent throughout their lives.

The IQ of the child is generally not reliably determined until he or she is of elementary school age, so most parents of infants will only know that their child seems to react or learn slowly. Physicians generally agree that mild mental retardation is impossible to diagnose within the first year. Unless there is an obvious genetic defect, such as Down's syndrome, even moderate and severe mental retardation may not be detected for months or years, depending on how observant the parents are.

Several signs indicate risk for mental retardation, though most of the infants at risk will not be mentally retarded. At risk factors include children from families with genetic disorders involving mental retardation, siblings of a retarded child, low socioeconomic status, age of mother (younger than 18 or older than 38) at the child's birth, use of certain drugs during pregnancy, presence of certain illnesses (e.g., rubella, toxemia, diabetes) during pregnancy, abnormally fast or prolonged labor, low Apgar score (which describes the child's physical adjustment to birth) five minutes after birth, abnormality in the placenta, convulsions after delivery, abnormally low birth weight, failure to regain birth weight within about ten days, and the presence of obvious birth defects.[6]

Usually parents begin to suspect that their child is retarded when he or she fails to keep pace with peers. The usual response is indecision about whether the child is normal. If the condition persists, the family takes the child to their physician, who will generally ask for the consultation of a specialist if he or she cannot rule out mental retardation.

If some conditions that could lead to mental retardation are caught early enough, the baby might not develop the retardation. For example, metabolic disorders such as phenylketonuria can be treated if caught early. Thyroid disorders are sometimes treatable depending on when the disorder began and other factors.

Decisions about the care of the child will begin early in the child's life. Testing can establish the likelihood that the child will be able to succeed in public school programs. In cases of profound mental retardation, the family might have to decide whether to institutionalize the child permanently, institutionalize the child part time or for specific training, or handle all child care at home. Often the family begins to raise the child at home and continues unless they discover that they cannot cope with the demands of rearing a handicapped child. Other reactions of families to handicapped children are discussed in a later section of this chapter.

MINIMAL BRAIN DYSFUNCTION

Minimal brain dysfunction is a catchall term that describes learning, perceptual, or behavioral difficulties that are thought to have resulted from injury, immaturity, or malfunction of the central nervous system. Damage is thought to be localized, so that the child might appear normal in most respects but experience difficulty in a limited area—such as being unable to understand what is heard, being hyperkinetic or overly aggressive, to name a few.

Usually, the child develops emotional difficulties as a secondary problem. This is thought to be due to the reactions of others in the child's environment. Avoidance, rejection, or even hostility toward the child shape the child's behavior to be even more objectionable and creates a cycle of rejection.

Boys outnumber girls about six to one in incidence of minimal brain dysfunction.[7] Usually, minimal brain dysfunction will not be detected until the elementary or middle school years. Once the diagnosis is made, parents often feel relief of guilt about their parenting skills. The tendency (and danger) is, then, to depend for primary treatment mainly on drugs and to avoid parental responsibility for working with the child on the behavioral difficulties and social and emotional development.

PHYSICAL HANDICAPS

Physical handicaps may be relatively mild, such as club foot—which occurs in one of every three hundred births—and congenital hip dislocation, which occurs from one to two times per one thousand births. Or the effect may be relatively serious, such as with spina bifida (protrusion of spinal nerves through the spinal cord), which occurs in three of every one thousand births, or congenital heart defects which to some degree affect up to 1 percent of all babies in the United States.[8] There are so many congenital physical defects that it would be impossible to list them. The defining characteristics are that they limit the health and capabilities of the child and mobilize the family around the child to insure that adequate child and medical care is obtained.

Having a baby who has a physical deformity or defect is a great shock for the parents. Usually parents express anxiety about the health of their baby as the labor is progressing. Apgar and Beck[9] suggest that every expectant parent thinks about or prays for a healthy infant. In 93 percent of the births, the infant is healthy. In the other times, parents often feel initial shock and denial. "This can't happen to me," they think. They often want to escape, to run away.

At birth, physicians and nurses often want to spare the parents the pain of knowledge. They reassure the parents that "At least he has all his fingers and toes," when the child has club foot. Or they might say, "At least one of the twins is all right." Generally, the baby is quickly removed from the delivery room for care by the hospital staff. To the extent that parents are kept from seeing or handling their physically handicapped child or that they refuse to see or handle the child, the parents will have a difficult time accepting him or her as part of the family.[10] Parents must give up the image of a healthy child and mourn the loss of that image if they are to accept their child as a unique and valuable human being whom God has delivered to them for their care.

Often the acceptance of the birth-defective child is made

even more difficult by the social situation. Friends and relatives do not know whether to offer congratulations or condolences for the child. They often resolve their ambivalence by not visiting or calling, which deprives the family of needed social support during their adjustment. If they do visit, the friends and relatives often feel uncomfortable and stilted in their conversation. Parents also experience ambivalence and discomfort and are unsure of how to act or what to say to their friends and family. Sometimes the discomfort of friends persists after the infancy of the baby, which limits the parents' social contacts. Other responses of families to the physically handicapped child are discussed in a later section of this chapter.

CHRONIC ILLNESS IN THE CHILD

Chronic illness involves long-term care of the ill child, which is usually carried out by the family. In acute illness, the physician or hospital generally cares for the child, but the family does most of the care for the chronically ill child, except for times in which the illness shows acute exacerbations requiring intensive medical attention. Numerous disorders are subsumed under the label "chronic illness," including cystic fibrosis, cerebral palsy, myelomeningocele, diabetes, and asthma. Each disease involves unique medical treatment but, like mental retardation, minimal brain dysfunction, and congenital physical handicaps, chronic illnesses tend to share common effects on the family.

Some of the demands of chronic illness on the family differ from other disorders. With the chronically ill child, the family must live near medical facilities that can treat the child's illness. Regular care of the child often involves compliance with medical regimens that are complicated and noxious. For example, children with cystic fibrosis might be required to take over fifty pills, engage in exercise, and adhere to other therapies that might involve two or more hours *each day.* Because children (and adults too) simply get tired of the constant attention even to life-maintaining medical discipline, compliance with the medical routine is difficult.

The family of the chronically ill child also experiences recurrent grief, as the child reaches developmental milestones and cannot function normally.[11] Because most chronic

193

illnesses affect the child's life expectancy, the family lives with the constant knowledge that the child might die suddenly. Despite their efforts to live so that they enjoy the child while he or she is alive, the thoughts of anticipatory grief are frequently in the minds of the parents. Other decisions are affected by this ambiguity. Career advancement might be affected if a company wished to transfer a parent to an area where medical attention is not readily available. Finally, medical expenses required to care for the chronically ill child are often staggering, and families can invest enormous energy in trying to find financial relief from the government or from private foundations and organizations. Additional financial burdens can cause strains on the family if parents have to work long hours or two jobs in addition to the additional caretaking tasks required of the parents.

COMMON EFFECTS ON THE FAMILY OF MENTAL RETARDATION, PHYSICAL HANDICAP, AND CHRONIC ILLNESS OF A CHILD

Patterson and McCubbin have identified nine categories of hardships experienced by families of children requiring special care.[12]

1. Strained family relationships. Parents are often overprotective of the child which inhibits the child's independence. Coalitions between the primary caretaker—usually the mother—and the child can create power struggles and children who act out. In addition, siblings might feel unwanted or unfavored, thus resenting their handicapped sibling. Blaming might be common.

Both the child and the parent who is thought to be genetically responsible might be blamed. The child might be rejected by parents, siblings, and even outsiders. Worry and resentment about the caretaking responsibilities of the parents might characterize family relationships. Siblings might compete for parental time or attention and they might be compared with the handicapped child. Marital relationships can also be strained.

2. Modifications of family activities and goals. The demands of child care and the requirement of staying near medical

treatment facilities might curtail vacation, leisure, career, and other family plans.

3. Increased tasks and commitments.

4. Increased financial burdens.

5. Need for housing adaptation. This might require limitations in the location of housing and might also involve modifications to the house to include wheelchair access or other special features.

6. Social isolation. Because of the additional tasks of child-rearing and the extra financial burdens, families might withdraw from much social interaction. In addition, others might avoid the family because they are unsure of how to relate to the child.

7. Medical concerns.

8. Differences in school experiences. Special needs must often be met in the school environment. Classes for mentally retarded, visually impaired, or physically handicapped children often involve special attention of parents and assertive interaction with members of the school system.

9. Grieving.

These effects continue through the life of the child. There are different focuses as the child ages.[13] In pregnancy and early infancy, the major tasks of the parents are fourfold. (1) The initial crisis must be experienced and worked through. This will involve shock, grief for loss of the ideal, and acceptance of the baby as a unique and valued member of the family. (2) The family must procure thorough diagnostic services. This often involves uncertainty and effort for parents to meet the multitude of appointments. Some tests are intrusive for the infant, so the family must learn to withstand seeing the child in discomfort. (3) The family must adjust to the intensive medical treatment of the child once the disorder is diagnosed. This might involve learning to give injections, forcing the child to take medications while the child struggles to avoid them, and performing other tasks that the child cannot understand and does not enjoy. (4) The parents must work through their understanding of God's role in their difficulties. Initially, the parents might blame God for afflicting them. At other times they might feel that God is punishing them for past or present sinful behavior. Parents might bargain with God and actively seek a supernatural healing. Over time, families shape their understanding of the problem and God's role in it. For some families, bitterness can rule their spiritual relationship. For others, chronic dissatisfaction with life and a fundamental distrust of God might be their resolution. For others, the problem is seen as a challenge with which to cope with reliance on God. For still others, the child can be looked at as a blessing that promotes spiritual growth among family members.

COPING WITH DIFFICULTY: TWO CASE STUDIES

"Two teenage girls and a retarded infant! What else could go wrong?" Chad Evert, 46-year-old executive, complained to his co-worker, Tom Needle, over lunch at the country club. "Bonnie is beside herself. She spends every minute of the day on that child, washing it, playing with it, talking with it. Frankly, I've just about had it. I'm about ready to put the kid into a home."

"Things sound as if they are really building up," said Tom.

"They've built up. I am so mad I could spit. We should have known better. We thought menopause was over, but obviously it wasn't. It was so *dumb*. We had been so fortunate with the girls. Even though Bonnie's family had a history of mental retardation, we didn't really think that it would happen to us. We should have known. Should have known." He shook his head.

"What are you doing about it?"

"There's nothing to do. Just put up with it," Chad exploded. "The kid's physically as healthy as a horse. He'll probably live to be a hundred, and Bonnie and I will grow old caring for him." Chad ran his hand through his thinning hair. "I'm sorry. I know that sounds harsh. But sometimes I feel *angry*. It sounds stupid, but it just isn't fair."

"You sound as if you are blaming God."

"Well, wouldn't you? My conception of God has done a remarkable turnaround in the last year and a half. I used to see him as kind and loving, but now . . . I don't know. He must enjoy seeing us suffer. Now, wait. Don't give me any lecture. I know in my head that he is supposed to be loving, but it is different now."

"It sure has made a difference in your work, Chad. I've noticed that since the baby was born, you have seemed to have no energy, and have seemed to have a chip on your shoulder. I know that's hard to hear, but. . . ."

"Well, I feel so mad all the time now. I'm mad at the kid. And I know he didn't make himself retarded on purpose. I'm angry at Bonnie for being the carrier of defective genes. I'm angry at the physicians for not being able to do anything and for charging so much money to do nothing except take up more time to run another ten tests. My anger just runs out of me onto about everyone and everything I see or do. You asked what I'm doing about it. I'm doing nothing. I'm just hoping to survive."

The Donaldson Family

Chad Evert looked at the man across from him. John Donaldson had agreed to meet with Chad for lunch three days after they had become acquainted through Tom, their mutual friend. Tom had suggested that Chad meet the Donaldsons, who had a four-year-old child with cerebral palsy. The Everts had gotten together with the Donaldsons and the Needles for dinner and although the evening had been largely lighthearted and happy, the talk had turned to the difficulties of rearing handicapped children at several points. Chad had been impressed with the quiet faith of the Donaldsons—especially John's. He was a mail carrier, whose financial status was certainly not as secure as Chad's who received a large executive salary; yet he seemed to believe that his needs were being met sufficiently. There was no trace of the bitterness and anger that Chad had felt so often lately.

Now as the two men sat together, Chad asked John, "How do you do it? How do you stay so calm about all that you must have gone through with your child?"

"Our child? You mean Patti, the one with cerebral palsy. The other three don't really cause quite the comment."

"Other *three*?! I didn't know you had any others."

197

"We have four altogether—twelve, nine, six, and four. After Patti, we decided we had better stop, though. We had originally hoped for five, but it was just a little too much work after Patti came."

"How do you handle four? We are absolutely overwhelmed with three."

"We have our moments," John said. "Especially within the first year. The first year was quite an adjustment. After a very depressing year, though, we got ourselves together and got some perspective on things. That helped."

"What kind of perspective?"

"Well, I was complaining to my pastor one night after an elders meeting and he talked to me pretty straight. He asked if I thought that I was the only person who had ever had any difficulties. He said I sounded like the people C. S. Lewis had talked about in an essay, that instead of God being on the judgment seat and us on trial, modern humans had assumed the judgment seat and placed God in the dock.[14] We had him on trial. Well, that was not exactly what I wanted to hear. But it was what I needed to hear. I didn't want to be in the position of judging God."

"How did that help?"

"It didn't at first. In fact, I got pretty angry with my pastor."

"But it helped later?"

"Yeah. It convicted me that God had not organized the universe for my pleasure. That's what I had been accusing God of—not considering my pleasure."

"That's a hard way of looking at it." Chad rubbed his hand over his head.

"I discovered that I had been angry with God for making life tough for me. That showed a basic mistrust of God's purposes. When I looked back over my entire life, I realized that he had always had my growth and my character at heart. Not everything he did for me was for my pleasure. I had this revelation one day when I was disciplining my oldest boy. He was about nine at the time. He had gone over to the neighbor's house to play and they had decided that they absolutely *had* to see the rock quarry about two miles from the house. Off they went. Unfortunately, they did not have the sense of direction to find the quarry. They got lost. I found them two hours later, wandering around in the hills behind our house. They didn't see anything wrong with the experience. They thought it was an adventure."

"I would have spanked them good for that."

"I did. There I was, in the middle of a spanking, with my hand upraised. Johnny was crying. I was talking to him in between spankings, telling him that I loved him and that if I didn't love him I would just let him do whatever he wanted and would never make life tough on him. Suddenly I just froze, for I realized that God was doing the same thing with me."

"You mean punishing you? With an ill child?"

"Not exactly. He was giving us something that would build our character in later times. He was giving us trials, so we could overcome them with his help."

"That's kind of rough on Patti, isn't it?" Chad asked. "Making her have cerebral palsy to teach you a little lesson."

"That's an interesting way of putting it. I guess when I look back now and see the easy-going way that I was coasting away from God, it doesn't seem like a *little* lesson. It seems like a pretty important lesson for me."

"But still, honestly, the idea of using a little girl and making her suffer just to teach you a lesson. That doesn't sit right."

"I guess I don't look at it quite like that. God is more concerned about our ultimate character than our temporary pleasure. I think he also is more concerned about Patti's character than her pleasure. Through her cerebral palsy, she has learned many wonderful lessons. She has learned the meaning of dependency on God and on others. She has learned that life is a gift, not a right, and that she should be grateful for the gift. She has developed a trust in God that is fully evident even at four years of age. In Romans 8, it says that the sufferings of this time are not worth comparing with the glory to come. That is the lesson that her disease has taught everyone in our family— not just at an intellectual level but at the very day-to-day level where we live."

"That's an important lesson all right. But I have a hard time with it."

"Like I say, so did I at first," said John. "I don't look at it as being any great accomplishment on my part. After all, God engineered the session where I had my big insight."

"You put a lot of trust in God controlling everything."

"After I got my mind changed around, it did seem that I could see his hand in most things."

Chad looked thoughtfully at John. "Well, I'm not there yet. Maybe you can pray for me. I know that I would like to have that assurance. Right now, the circumstances just seem to point me in other ways."

"How are those ways leading?"

"They are not leading me any closer to God. But that's the way I see it, anyway."

AN ANALYSIS

There are other aspects of coping with a child with a long-term impairment. Why did I choose to focus on the person's spiritual perspective? A number of independent studies have suggested that a person's faith is crucial to effective coping. For example, Shere found that maintaining hope and attachment is important for good social-emotional development of a family and children with cerebral palsy.[15] Cardwell suggested that critical ingredients in handling cerebral palsy are *faith*, optimism, and courage.[16] Darling studied families in which one or more child had a birth defect.[17] An altruistic approach to the problem, agape love, was found to describe the families who coped well.

Chodoff, Friedman, and Hamburg examined parents of children with malignant diseases and observed that most parents who effectively coped with the disease had searched and found some broad religious framework in which to understand the disease.[18] In summary, one of the chief difficulties in dealing with an illness or chronic problem of an infant will be the family's understanding of the meaning of the tragedy. Their faith, or lack of trust in God, will be important in how the family ultimately handles the difficulty.

In a major study of parents of chronically ill children, Mc-Cubbin, McCubbin, Nevin, and Cauble (1979) found that the coping attempts of parents fell into three broad categories:[19]

1. Maintaining family integration, i.e., (working together

as a family), cooperation, and an optimistic definition of the situation.

2. Maintaining social support and relationships, self-esteem, and psychological stability (through engaging in activities "for themselves").

3. Understanding the medical situation through communication with other parents and consultation with medical personnel.

Studying over five hundred families of children with cerebral palsy, cystic fibrosis, or myelomeningocele, McCubbin, McCubbin, Patterson, Cauble, Wilson, and Warwick [20] found that each of the coping patterns had different effects on the family for mothers and for fathers.

Mothers' coping strategies of maintaining family integration, cooperation, and optimism promoted family cohesiveness. The same coping strategies when used by fathers promoted family cohesiveness too, but also reduced conflict and promoted organization within the family. Mothers' supportiveness, attempts at esteem-building, and efforts at maintaining psychological stability were associated with family expressiveness. Fathers' use of those strategies was not related systematically to any family variables. Mothers' use of medical communication was related to family cohesiveness, while fathers' use of medical information related to family control. This study demonstrated that mothers and fathers used the same ways of handling situations, but mothers' efforts at coping were related to the emotional environment within the family while fathers' coping strategies were related to the functioning of the family. Both parents were necessary for effective family coping with the long-term childhood problems.

COUNSELING FAMILIES WITH CHRONIC PROBLEMS

Generally, families will cope more or less effectively with their difficulties. Counselors can best help families to use effective coping mechanisms rather than ineffective ones. In addition, the father and the mother should both be encouraged to participate in family coping. Counseling should generally be confined to providing information that helps the family deal with the specific problem, guiding family members to find appropriate social support groups and resources, and assisting them with understanding where the difficulty fits into the overall scheme of their spiritual lives.

Counseling should be oriented toward solving problems and changing the perceptions of situations. It should avoid delving into the past of family members. If the counselor sticks with specific difficulties and tries to help the family solve those difficulties, he or she will usually achieve more success with the family than if attempts were made to do traditional individual or family therapy.

Generally, counseling should concentrate on prevention of secondary difficulties arising from the medical problem. Providing ongoing support groups and maintaining a list of resources about how to cope with the difficulties are the best means of prevention.

CHAPTER NINE

UNEXPECTED MIDLIFE PREGNANCIES

CLINT AND ANN HAD HAD A ROUGH TIME with their child-rearing. They had four children and made no secret of their feelings that they should have stopped with three. Fortunately, they had been careful in the family never to mention that feeling to their youngest child. Their family had begun early, when Clint and Ann were both in college. At nineteen for Clint and eighteen for Ann, they had married and become pregnant almost immediately. They had made sacrifice after sacrifice for the children throughout their twenties and thirties. Now, the oldest daughter was married, the oldest son was in the army, and the number three child, a daughter, was almost ready to graduate from college. Rob was the only child now living at

203

home. He was a senior in high school who seemed destined to attend the state university on a track scholarship. Clint and Ann were forty-nine and forty-eight, respectively.

Ann had developed endometriosis at forty-two, and began to show signs of menopause five years later. They had discontinued birth control measures shortly after she became forty-eight, and they settled down to await their "freedom" from children.

"It seems as though our entire life has been spent raising children," Ann said after they were told she was pregnant again.

The physician explained their "options," by which he meant that they should seriously consider an abortion. When they refused, he suggested that Ann undergo an amniocentesis test. He explained the dangers of retardation, birth defects, and poor health for mother and child when the mother is over 40. Clint and Ann were resolute. "Why should we have an amniocentesis?" they said. "We don't believe in abortion, so what good would it do?"

"But if we do an amniocentesis," argued the physician, "we can tell if the child has genetic defects. We can prevent needless suffering by the child and also by you. I know that the child will be a difficult and stressful adjustment for the two of you. If it is retarded or deformed, its quality of life will be so low that it is a service to end the pregnancy."

"I'm sorry, doctor," said Clint. "We just don't see things your way. We both feel that life is sacred. It is given by God and is not something for us to choose to end because we somehow don't think the child will have a high quality of life. The way we see it, compared to God, even the intelligence of an Einstein or the physical capabilities of an Olympic champion are minuscule. How do we, then, presume that because a baby does not measure up to our intelligence or our standards of physical capability that somehow its life is not valuable? We believe that God has given this pregnancy for a purpose. We don't understand his purpose right now. And it seems absolutely overwhelming to think about raising another child after we thought our family was complete. But we trust God, and we will search for his purpose and not presume to take a life he has considered important enough to create."

Clint and Ann decided to seek the assistance of a different obstetrician for care throughout the pregnancy. Ann spent most of the pregnancy depressed. That summer, after eight months, Ann went into labor and gave birth to a baby boy whom they named Jeff. The birth was particularly long and difficult and Jeff's Apgar score was low at birth and five minutes post-partum.

Clint was outside the nursery when he noticed that the nurses were all around the isolette housing Jeff. That evening Jeff died. Ann, still feeling the depression she experienced throughout the pregnancy, talked to the pastor.

"Father Jim, I know I have killed my son," she cried. "My depression created an environment that he knew was not good for him. I feel so guilty."

Her pastor answered. "Ann, you've experienced a terrific loss. I know of so little that I can say to comfort you. I do know though that God's hand is in your life and in Clint's. God knows that despite the hardships, you would gladly have loved and cared for your new son. You have been faithful parents for almost thirty years. God did not take Jeff because there was no love in your family."

"Why, then? Why? Why did we have to go through this terrible ordeal? For nothing? Our baby *died*. Today, after Jeff died, I looked out the window and saw the gorgeous blue sky. I thought of the beautiful green of the grass and the palms waving in the ocean breeze. I thought of the waves breaking on the beach. And I thought that Jeff would never be able to enjoy any of that with me. I couldn't see him swimming, or playing tennis, or doing school work. He was dead."

"Ann," the minister continued, "death is certainly a terrible loss, and you need to grieve that loss. You have lost the sight of Jeff's development and growth. You have lost the joys and struggles that you would have gone through trying to raise Jeff to be a man of God. But you know as I do that death is not the worst thing that can happen to a Christian. Life will continue after death and perhaps you will be reunited as a family with God some day."

"I know. I remember how you told me that when my mother died. And it helps. I have thought about taking my

205

own life all day. I have just felt like I'm ready to go—the pain is too much. It is only the thought of maybe denying myself that meeting with the Lord that has held me together. But it is such a grief."

Clint and Ann experienced a later-life pregnancy that ended tragically. Others move from pregnancy into a second parenthood or perhaps a first parenthood. Their struggles last longer, though Clint and Ann are likely to experience grief for years over loss of their infant.[1] If the later-life pregnancy is unexpected and unwanted—at least at first—the adjustment will likely be difficult. Having a child in later life disrupts established lives and adds to numerous other life events in many circumstances.

OTHER TASKS OF MIDLIFE

Like Clint and Ann, many couples nearing the end of their childbearing years will have a family that they feel is the right size or even a little too large for comfort. Many will already have begun to launch their children, but others will have children who are all at home. The addition of the newborn into a household that is already strained with many child-care activities can add to the stress of the birth of the child.

On the other hand, older children can help the couple with many child-care responsibilities. One danger is that the eldest sibling might be vested with too much responsibility without any authority to raise the child. The younger siblings can become organized around the oldest child, often called the "parental child." If this difficulty occurs, parents must correct the power structure and assume the responsibility for child care that belongs to them, placing the eldest child back in the role of child. Then the parents can move to having the eldest child handle some tasks under their definite supervision.

Another stress faced by midlife parents who are completing their childbearing years when they become pregnant is the presence of teenage children in the home. When a child enters the teen years, the parents often experience many conflicts. The teen begins to undergo dramatic physical changes. Boys experience changes in their bodily structure as their physique matures. They sprout facial hair and their voice changes. Girls begin to menstruate, their breasts develop, and their bodies become more curvacious.

All these physical changes are visible reminders to the parents that the parents are aging. Their bodies are changing, too. They seem to be injured simply by tying their shoes. The man might suffer from the "furniture disease" in which the chest falls into the drawers. The woman might gain weight, develop multicolored places behind the knees and at the ankles, and have skin that droops.

"Why can't I get older in peace?" one middle-aged parent wailed. "Every day my adolescent comes in and reminds me that I'm not getting any younger."

Sexuality is also on the minds of most adolescents and their parents. The adolescent is just becoming aware of his or her sexual identity while the parent is becoming aware that his or her sexual identity is more fragile than once believed. Teens wrestle with self-control of a strong drive while parents often experience a waning in their sexual drive. Some parents, as they experience this change, strive to maintain their illusion of youth by initiating extra-marital sexual encounters or by changing their sexual behavior with their spouses by trying exotic positions or behaviors. Both teens and parents are wrestling with issues in the same areas, so teens keep the issues on the parents' minds.

Career motivation is also usually awakening for the teen. He or she is making decisions about an initial career. Courses are planned and decisions are made about whether, where, or when to attend college. Simultaneously, parents might reevaluate their career identity. The mother might have dedicated her early years of marriage to childrearing and she is intent on entering the work force and making a contribution to society through work. Men might have tried to achieve fulfillment through their efforts at work and, having become dissatisfied with their ability to achieve lasting satisfaction, they might be thinking of a career change. Or they may be contemplating ways to decrease their work involvement and increase their involvement with family, friends, and church. With teens and parents dealing with the same issues, parents are constantly reminded of their struggles.

Besides the many personal issues that are salient for the midlife couple, their marriage satisfaction is generally at a lower ebb than at earlier times in their lives together. For men who are happily married, marriage satisfaction is lowest when children are in adolescence; satisfaction improves again when children begin to leave home. For men who are not happily married, marriage satisfaction generally continues to decline as the children begin to leave home and throughout the retirement years.

For women who are happily married, marriage satisfaction is generally lower when their children are in adolescence than in earlier times of the marriage. However, when children begin to leave home, women experience still further reductions in their marriage satisfaction. A sense of satisfaction with the marriage again rises once the children have been "launched." For unhappily married women, marriage satisfaction—like their spouses'—tends to decrease continually after the onset of children.

Finally, parents' expectations are important. If the couple is eagerly anticipating time when they will not have child-care duties, they will find the unexpected midlife pregnancy unpleasant and their adjustment will likely be long and difficult.

RISKS OF MIDLIFE PREGNANCIES

There are risks associated with any pregnancy, but they dramatically increase as the parents age. One problem that is increased with the age of the mother is early pregnancy loss. It has been estimated that from 15 to 25 percent of all pregnancies are miscarried in women in the United States.[2] It is difficult to know how accurate this figure is because very early pregnancies are often not recognized as pregnancies. Generally, the spontaneous miscarriage occurs because the infant is physically malformed and would likely not survive birth anyway. Other early pregnancy losses occur because the mother has damaged the fallopian tubes through pelvic inflammatory disease, the use of contraceptives, or through some other disease. With the fallopian tubes damaged, the likelihood of an ectopic pregnancy is increased; mothers older than forty have increased risk of ectopic pregnancies.[3]

Other common problems in older women are fibroid tumors and endometriosis. Fibroid tumors are benign growths in the uterus that may range in size up to the size of a softball. Generally, fibroid tumors are of concern only if they grow quite large or result in excessive bleeding during menstruation. Endometriosis is caused by cells of the lining of the uterus (endometrium) attaching themselves to other places in the pelvic cavity, such as the ovaries, or the fallopian tubes. These cells can block implantation from occurring and cause other problems. Although the cause of endometriosis is unknown, it has been found in high incidence with career women who have deferred parenthood.[4]

Other medical problems can occur with pregnancy if the mother has an ongoing medical condition such as hypertension, vascular disease, kidney disease, diabetes, or abnormalities in the reproductive system. All of the above disorders increase in frequency with the age of the mother. Generally, these conditions make it more difficult for the baby to receive the nutrients it needs for growth, or the environment is risky for normal growth. Normal births are usually possible despite the presence of these disorders in the adults *if* the pregnancy is carefully monitored by medical personnel and *if* the mother maintains a healthy lifestyle.

There is also an increased likelihood that the midlife pregnancy will produce twins or other multiple births. For example, the chances that a mother under thirty will have a multiple birth are less than one in one hundred; the chances of a mother between thirty and thirty-five having a multiple birth are one in seventy-five; and for a mother between thirty-five and forty, her chances for multiple births are one in sixty-five.[5] After age forty, the chances are reduced to about one in one hundred again. Although the family might not consider the multiple pregnancy to be a problem in itself, multiple births have more complications—the babies are born prematurely, and such births result in babies who die or are handicapped more often than is true of single births.[6]

There are other medical risks that occur infrequently, yet still affect older mothers more often than younger mothers. For instance, placenta praevia is more likely in older mothers than in younger mothers. This occurs when the placenta attaches low on the uterine wall or even over the cervix. The likelihood is high with this condition that the placenta, which supplies nutrients from the mother to the baby, will become damaged or detached and the baby will receive inadequate nutrients to sustain its life. The same effect might occur in the event of intrauterine growth retardation, in which the placenta fails to develop adequately.[7] Finally, older mothers have prolonged or difficult labors more often than younger mothers.[8]

In addition to increased medical risks throughout pregnancy, women over thirty-five have a larger risk of delivering by a Caesarean birth.[9] Despite the increased risks associated with births to mothers over thirty-five, most mothers deliver their children without difficulty. The risk of complications in pregnancy and delivery are reduced markedly if the mother is in good shape physically and has eaten nutritionally throughout the pregnancy. Most obstetricians who deliver babies to mothers of all ages believe that the physical condition of the mother is more important than age.[10] Complications are also reduced if the mother does not smoke or drink alcohol during the pregnancy.[11]

Risk to the Baby

Older mothers have somewhat increased chances of having babies with congenital deformities, probably because disorders such as diabetes and hypertension are increasingly likely with the increased age of the parent, and those disorders increase the risk that the baby will be malformed.

One of the few birth defects that are of chromosomal origin that increases with age is Down's syndrome. Down's syndrome involves an irregularity in the twenty-first chromosome—having three instead of the normal two. The syndrome produces an infant with mongoloid facial characteristics and, usually, profound mental retardation. As the mother ages, the risk of having a child with Down's syndrome increases markedly. At age 30, this risk is 1/885; at age 35, it is 1/365; at 40, it is 1/109; and at 45, it is 1/32.[12]

Because most people are aware of the increasing risk of having a child with Down's syndrome, many women who are pregnant in their forties will elect to have an amniocentesis. This procedure is not a benign procedure. It involves risk, to the mother and especially to the baby. An amniocentesis involves withdrawing amniotic fluid, which contains cells from the baby, from the uterus. Usually, the mother is pierced by a long needle which also punctures the amniotic sack containing the baby. The mother might be injured by the needle piercing her bowel or bladder or by infection. But the greater risk is to the infant. Infection or bruising might occur, and premature labor might even be induced.

A more serious threat is the condition when the baby's and the mother's blood types do not match. Such a condition might allow their circulations to mix, which could result in the mother's immune system rejecting the baby or at least killing fetal blood cells.

An even greater threat to the baby occurs if chromosomal irregularities are detected, which happens in almost 5 percent of the cases when the mother is over forty.[13] Of every one hundred women whose amniocentesis tests show chromosomal irregularities, ninety-four elect to abort their child.[14]

Other risks to the child occur after birth. Two of the most common are low birth weight, which is often a result of premature delivery, and perinatal death (from twenty-eight-weeks gestation through four-weeks postdelivery). Low birth weight occurs in about 6 percent of the births to mothers from twenty to twenty-nine, in about 7 percent of births to mothers of thirty to thirty-four, and in 9 to 10 percent to mothers thirty-five and over. Perinatal mortality occurs in about 2 to 3 percent of deliveries to mothers under thirty-five and 4 to 6 percent of deliveries to mothers over thirty-five.[15]

DEALING WITH STILLBIRTH, MISCARRIAGE, AND INFANT MORTALITY

Of every one hundred pregnancies, about one dies through stillbirth after the twentieth week of gestation. Because stillbirth and miscarriage happen within the mother's womb, one research team has called stillbirth "the invisible death."[16] The reality of the miscarriage or stillbirth is difficult to convey to outsiders. The baby is only a "concept" to relatives or friends.

To the parents, however, the baby *seems* alive after they feel it move.[17] Psychologically, they feel that the baby is their child, and they often report that the baby has a distinct personality from the first time they feel him or her move.

"Ronnie always was a kicker. He seemed never to have any room. He rolled over, then POW! That foot would come out. When he would be still, and I guess he was asleep, then I'd wake him by pushing him around. He'd immediately let me have it again. Boom! Right in the ribs." Sue described her son who was delivered stillborn.

Ron, Sue's husband, said, "I always wanted to coach soccer. I thought we had another Pele. Now he's not there. Just dead."

DeFrain[18] sent five hundred and fifty volunteers nationwide a ten-page survey with open-ended questions. Of those, three hundred and four returned completed surveys—80 percent mothers. All participants had lost children through stillbirth. The authors have written an emotionally moving and enlightening account of the responses of parents to stillbirth, keeping interpretation to a minimum. Most of the information in the following sections has been adapted from that book, which is recommended reading for both professionals and people who have experienced a stillbirth or miscarriage.

The Experience

The vast majority of parents found out that their baby had died before the delivery. For some, the time for preparation was helpful, allowing an adjustment before viewing the baby. For others, though, the knowledge that their baby was dead made the labor difficult. One woman said that the labor seemed like a cruel joke. She had a long and difficult labor and then at the end had only empty arms to show for it.

The initial reaction of most parents was shock. Some became hysterical when they found out about the death. Others felt numb. When Kirby and I found that we had miscarried our first baby, I felt sick. I wanted to throw up, but was not able to. I had a feeling of unreality in which I wanted to show grief because I thought I should experience it, but my body did not seem to want to cooperate. Other people have reported a dreamlike state as their initial reaction to the news of the death. A husband will often report a strong concern for the physical and emotional well-being of the wife.

Following the initial shock came blame. The reaction is a natural response of trying to find meaning in a painful situation. The target of the blame varied with the couples. Some blamed the doctor or the hospital, while others blamed God. Quite a few felt that God was punishing them. Many parents blamed themselves. Feelings of guilt were common but not experienced by everyone; however, within a month almost everyone had felt some sense of guilt. The guilt was often carried for years by some of the participants in DeFrain's study.

People reported getting over their guilt feelings as a result of the doctors' assurance that the death was not the fault of the parents, or occasionally, when receiving the report of the autopsy. More than half said that the assurance of God's goodness and the knowledge that the child's death was somehow in his will, despite their inability to understand how, helped them handle their guilt feelings.

Finally, the reality of coping with death was faced. The hardship of the financial costs of the hospital stay, the doctors' bills, and the funeral were seen as unpleasant reminders that the baby had died and that other harsh realities of life also had to be faced.

Coping with Loss

More than half of the parents saw their dead baby, and all of them reported they were glad that they had. Most of the parents who did not see the baby wished later that they had, for in not viewing the baby, they felt their grief had been prolonged. Even among the parents who saw the baby, many said that they wished they had held him or her, or held him or her longer, or taken pictures. "It hurts me to know that I never held my baby in my arms" was a common lament of parents.

Parents found several aspects of miscarriage or stillbirth difficult. Some said that the hardest part was coming home from the hospital with empty arms. For some mothers the most troubling part was when their milk came in. Usually fathers had trouble calling the relatives and telling people about the death. Some parents thought the funeral was the most difficult part, though most also cited it as an element that speeded their healing, for they could release the child to God's care.

Almost 90 percent named the baby and many even observed birthdates in future years. They had a clear sense that the baby was a real and an important part of their family. In our family, we often talk about how we will be reunited in heaven one day. Since our baby died early, the sex was never determined. Jonathan, surrounded by three sisters, sometimes says that he will someday perhaps have a brother to play with in heaven.

Many people tried to escape the pain of the death. Some in the group under study moved; almost half of the people moved within a year of their infant's death. For others, sleep was the respite they sought, though most reported that sleep did not help them cope with the loss. Still others sought escape through alcohol, and almost a quarter of the participants reported seriously considering suicide.

Generally, the greatest help in coping with the loss was the parents' social support network. The family, especially one's spouse, proved very important in helping adjust to the death. Other family members were also helpful—even the other children in the family. Parents within Christian communities often mentioned the church community as being of invaluable support. Church members helped through calling, visiting, and just being available when needed. In addition, it was not uncommon for church members to help the family by providing meals, doing housework, and caring for other children while the family got back together emotionally. Hugging was mentioned frequently as an important part of the community of faith. Pastors were frequently cited as being helpful, though the writers caution that "one superstar, heavily trained professional is not going to bring the grieving parent back to health. Rather, a loving community of people, all acting individually in their unique, kindly ways, will lead the bereaved back to emotional well-being."[19]

Coping with stillbirth is not instantaneous. The three hundred and four people surveyed reported that it took two or three years after the death before they were as happy as they were before the death. In addition, most families reported that their family life was disrupted substantially. The family life rebounded faster than the feelings of happiness of the individual parents, but it was still about one year before the shock waves of the child's death calmed within the family organization.

One Couple's Response

Reading a summary of the accounts of many families' experience of infant death can give a perspective about the many ways people experience and cope with their loss, but it cannot tell the depth of grief that is felt by individuals. Listen to one woman tell of her loss.

It was winter. There were no leaves on the trees. No baby robins chirping in the abandoned nest in the bush outside our window. We were ecstatic at finally conceiving a child after twenty years of marriage and about sixteen years of hoping and praying for a child. But then in the eighth month at our Lamaze class, the teacher could not find a heartbeat. That night, I went into labor and delivered Kelley Susan. Dead. I was devastated, hurt, angry. It seemed so unfair. We read of the millions of abortions; and then we are pregnant and our baby dies.

I wanted to be left alone. A nurse came into my recovery room. Both Will and I were crying together. The nurse didn't really ask. She just brought Kelley over to me, wrapped in a soft blanket, and placed her in my arms. She was so beautiful, but her color was bad because she had apparently been dead for a few days. I remember looking at her peaceful face and seeing my tears fall on her skin. I hugged her to me and felt a giant cavern within me that I thought could never be filled. Will had come to stand beside the bed and was looking down at our daughter. I never would know Kelley's laugh. Will and I would never go through the anxiety of waiting on her to come home from her first single date. I hugged her tight to my body and then asked Will if he wanted to hold her.

He took her lifeless little body in his strong hairy arms and wept aloud. It almost broke my heart.

We kept Kelley with us for a couple of hours, taking turns holding her. I knew that the Lord was good. I didn't understand his purpose, but I understood that he had given me an experience that would affect me from that moment on. I was a mother.

I thought of the women in my life. Mary, the mother of Jesus. She saw her son killed before her eyes. Mother Teresa. My first grade Sunday school teacher, Marge Cowper. All of these women had affected my life profoundly. I knew too that Kelley had affected me equally. My faith in God had been tested and strengthened and Will and I had shared another experience that would bond us together even more tightly. Our lives are not just important because of the years we live, but because of the impact we have on others. Kelley had had an impact on her world, and she was an important human whom God had graced us to parent for a few hidden months.

At the funeral, we had a celebration that God had taken Kelley to him, for we had prayed for Kelley from conception that the Holy Spirit would be active in her life and would create from the instant of conception a child who knew Jesus. After the funeral service, we had the casket opened and invited those who wanted to view Kelley before we placed her body in the cold December ground to await her resurrection in the end times.

A dear friend, Sharon Monroe, who had also lost a child during her pregnancy years earlier, gave me a moment to remember that typifies the sensitivity and love that our friends in the church showed us. She walked by the casket and gazed lovingly at Kelley as we stood by. Then, she took an infant's sweater—one that had been given her for her infant that had died—and spread it tenderly across Kelley. When I looked up from my tears, it had begun to snow outside.

ADVANTAGES TO HAVING BABIES IN MIDLIFE

Besides the risks and costs to having babies after forty, there are some distinct advantages.[20] Usually parents in their forties are on more solid financial footing than couples in their teens. The extra cushion of savings can relieve some anxiety about the future of the child. It can also free the parents to spend more time with their baby. Many people in their forties and beyond are less engrossed in advancing their careers than the thirty-year-old rising star of the corporation. They have moved beyond the stage of making a name for themselves and have begun to mentor younger members in their career field. The tendency to be a workaholic is lessened, and parents are often more available for the special events of childhood and adolescence.

In addition, the couple in their forties have generally arrived at a stable and relatively secure self-concept relative to couples in their twenties. They have simply seen more of life and tend to be less "thrown" by the ups and downs of living. The greater maturity can show up in the child-care and child-raising decisions made by the parents. In addition, the later birth often comes to parents who have raised other children. The parents are, then, experienced parents—which means they are usually free to make *other* mistakes in raising the baby, and not the same ones they made with earlier children.

COUNSELING FAMILIES WITH MIDLIFE PREGNANCIES

The couple who find that they are about to have a late pregnancy will generally not be interested in information about the birth. Most couples will have been through births previously and will feel confident about that aspect of the coming experience.

Some couples might require help in decision making, especially if they are considering an abortion. The salience of abortion as a political issue in our country has raised the consciousness of couples who might have previously considered abortion an easy solution to their difficulty. Now, they will often want to talk about their decision to gain the support of a professional for the decision they intend to make. Other couples might be firmly convinced that abortion is wrong, and then find that they are faced with a pregnancy in which the child is likely deformed or has Down's syndrome. Often this can shake their beliefs. What was once an academic commitment not to have an abortion might take on added emphasis when the decision stares them in the face.

As a counselor, you will help them arrive at a decision that they will be able to live with. Your guidance can be crucial as you help them examine the long- and short-term consequences of each decision.

Other couples might seek information from you about the risks of pregnancy. Usually, couples obtain such information from physicians (along with the values of the physicians). As you discuss the implications of pregnancy with the couple, you can gently probe to find how extensive and accurate their knowledge is. You might be able to enrich their knowledge base by sharing from your personal experience or from information gained through reading (see Appendix 5 for a list of recommended readings).

Often the couple might seek your help because they are concerned about the impact of a new birth on an already strained relationship between them and their older children. You might be able to help them learn new ways of handling their older children. A library of books about parenting adolescents and other children can be a useful resource.

In addition, the couple might have some other midlife tensions. The issues of sexuality, career, and identity are all raised by a late pregnancy, which may activate midlife conflicts and prompt one or both of the prospective new parents to reevaluate important aspects of their lives.

Usually, the couple in distress over a recently discovered pregnancy will need to talk about the difficulties they anticipate, to vent the emotion they are experiencing. However, after the emotion has declined, they can often be encouraged to examine the positive aspects of childbirth in later life. This might provide a valuable perspective that will serve to correct their perception of what they will experience.

Skills

Most of the skills that you are concerned with do not deal with the birth of the child directly. You might provide help with the difficulties of parenting adolescent children. Or you might provide help with handling any midlife conflict that arises with the discovery of the pregnancy. Finally, you might assist the woman, through counseling her on health habits and risks associated with alcohol, smoking, or being in poor condition physically.

Support

As the DeFrain study[21] pointed out, when helping parents grieve the death of their baby, no single helper is likely to be able to nurse an emotionally distraught parent back to emotional health. Rather, the professional can best provide personal support by being available when needed. The professional must be sensitive to the desires and needs of the couple while continuing to be true to his or her own beliefs.

For example, some couples become angry at God when their baby is stillborn. When the counselor speaks of God's will, the couple might be very blunt and turn their anger on the professional. Professionals must take care in how they express themselves, carefully feeling out the couple to determine their beliefs about the will of God in the child's death. If counselors find that the couple does not view the death as being within God's will, they might express the idea in a less direct form, such as: "I know that right now you are sad and angry about the death of your son. And I know, too, that it is impossible for you to see God's hand in this right now. From my perspective, though, I think that God has something for you to learn in this experience. I don't know exactly what it is or when you might discover it, but I know that God is good and has been good to you in the years I have known you and I am glad that Jesus is the same yesterday, today, and forever. I don't understand the why of this death, but I pray that the Lord will show you his will for you in handling this."

An important thing the professional, friend, or family member can do is provide assurance of God's goodness, omnipotence, and wisdom. The trial can help the couple grow in faith if they seek the Lord. This is one of the ministries of the professional—to help people in pain grow closer to God instead of farther away.

PREVENTION

Generally, midlife pregnancies are a result of the misjudgment of when the woman is past her fertility period. The best preventive measure is to continue to practice whatever birth control method is appropriate for the couple until they are absolutely assured that pregnancy is not possible.

Once the pregnancy occurs, the counselor can help the couple avoid some of the problems that are possible through warning the couple of the likely difficulties and counseling them to avoid potential troublesome behavior.

CHAPTER TEN

COUNSELING THE INFERTILE COUPLE

I ASK MY CLASSES AT VIRGINIA COMMONWEALTH UNIVERSITY what makes people depressed. Usually they arrive at an impressive list of situations that lead to depression. Almost invariably one of the reasons someone offers is "finding out you can't have kids when you want them." Usually, that is followed in short order by "finding out you can have kids when you don't want them." Throughout much of the book we have discussed the second option. But let us now look at the mirror image— counseling childless couples, the ultimate in a late-occurring pregnancy.

One difficulty in writing about infertility is that little research has been done concerning it. Ralph and Anne Martin

Matthews have written several reviews of the research and popular literature about infertility.[1] In one review, in late 1986,[2] they said

> References to infertility and involuntary childlessness are simply not found in most of the leading textbooks dealing with family life. . . . The rare text that does mention that subject usually limits its discussion to a brief consideration of the possibility of adoption as an alternative to biological parenthood . . . or to a discussion of alternative technologies of conception, such as artificial insemination. . . . No analysis of the social and psychological dimensions of involuntary childlessness is provided. Much the same can be said of the popular press. . . . The only literature that deals with social and social-psychological aspects of infertility and involuntary childlessness is based on the work of clinicians.

THE PROBLEM

Infertility is defined as the inability to achieve pregnancy within a stipulated period of time.[3] The length of the period of time differs with the culture. In some cultures, failure to achieve pregnancy within two years of marriage is grounds for divorce,[4] but in the United States, medical personnel usually do not consider there to be grounds for infertility testing unless the couple has tried for at least one year without success. Couples might define themselves as infertile in shorter or longer lengths of time than one year.

Many times, only the husband and wife know they are infertile. Few couples walk around telling others, "I'm infertile," though their difficulties often become public knowledge if they announce that they are trying to have children and they do not soon become pregnant.

The incidence of infertility is difficult to estimate, but has been variously placed at between 10 and 20 percent of all couples in the United States at any given time.[5] Many of those infertile couples are not sterile (permanently infertile), but the distress and anxiety experienced by couples unable to conceive is similar regardless of whether or not the difficulty ever is remedied.

We usually assume couples are fertile. The infertile couple can thus be hurt by the comments of well-meaning friends and relatives, because their infertility is hidden. In addition, the experience of infertility and the subjugation of the infertile couple to medical attempts to solve the problem can result in discomfort, hurt, frustration, and indignity. Parents can apply pressure on the couple to have offspring, and even the church, which has a generally pronatalist stand and whose activities are often oriented for family fun, can pressure them.

Infertility is difficult to cope with. When a woman is pregnant, everyone knows—before too long. The transition to parenthood is clearly marked by visible signs. When a man and woman are infertile, it is difficult for anyone to know. The boundaries of the transition are vague. The husband and wife must first undergo a period of instability: Can we or can we not have children? When they finally discover that they are sterile and that nothing can be done about it, profound loss is experienced. Yet the loss does not involve something that is seen— such as when a baby dies. It involves the loss of a potential. Grief is hard to experience because the loss is intangible. Yet the loss is painful and real and involves a large reordering of self-concepts and marital goals.

STAGES OF INFERTILITY AND STERILITY

Stigger has identified stages through which couples pass when they are infertile or sterile.[6] The first stage begins in childhood. Everyone is born to a parent and most children grow up in families. The natural assumption of almost all children is that they can become parents when they grow into adulthood. Most teenagers develop their sexual identities assuming that they can have children. Discussion often centers around how to *prevent* having children in the teen years and the need to remain a virgin and have children *later,* after marriage to the partner whom God has chosen for the teenager.

When marriage occurs, the newly wedded couple will usually be encouraged by their friends and family to put off having children in their first year or years of marriage to give the relationship time to grow and to negotiate the transition to marriage. In all these instances, fertility is assumed.

Finally, when the man and woman are ready for children, they might discontinue whatever birth control method they are practicing and actively try to conceive. Time passes, with no pregnancy.

Defending the Assumption

Everyone makes assumptions about the nature of life. When these assumptions are challenged by circumstances, we do not easily change the assumptions, even in the face of strong contradictory evidence. At first, we defend the assumption. Stigger identifies three phases of defense.[7] In the first phase, people deny that there is a problem. "Oh, there is nothing to be alarmed about. We've only been trying for three months." "Lots of couples take a while to become pregnant after they stop using birth control."

Initial denial is realistic. Assuming sexual intercourse twice weekly and good health of the spouses, only half of the couples will conceive within six months, and only 80 percent will conceive within a full year. Initial denial allows the couple to wait with little anxiety.

However, when they continue to try to conceive without success, they might move to the second phase of defense: acknowledging the presence of a problem but denying responsibility for the cause or cure of the problem. They might blame the doctor. Each spouse might blame the other. They might acknowledge that there is a problem and place it in God's hands, assuming that they are to do nothing except to continue regular sexual relations. Nonetheless, they cannot help but experience some frustration and anger. The anger might be undifferentiated and expressed out of proportion to any annoyance that occurs. It might show up as bickering between spouses, or as tension at work, or with in-laws.

The third phase of defense occurs when the man and woman begin to reason that if a problem exists, there must be a cure. The assumption of fertility is held tenaciously and they embark on a quest for a cure. Usually the home cure is tried first.

Coital and postcoital positions are manipulated. There is the pile-of-pillows beneath the hips coital position. Then, under the theory that gravity can be harnessed in the service of the couple, there is the balancing-on-the-shoulders position (post-coitus and sometimes during) and finally the balancing-on-the-shoulders-while-swinging-in-an-indoor-hammock (only for the very athletic). They emerge from home remedy attempts very tired (but in extremely good physical shape).

Feeling in peak condition, they consult a physician who introduces them to charts-and-graphs therapy. During this time, the wife takes her basal temperature several times a day. The husband might receive mysterious calls at work, after which he must rush home. After this, the man and woman might undergo testing by their physician and his or her learned cohorts. The woman might have her tubes blown, and the man might visit a doctor's office and be directed to provide a semen sample. Other more invasive tests might also be required.

Meanwhile, they begin to look more physically tired, not to mention anxious about the mechanical way their medical testing is going. Friends usually begin to offer emotional cures. Usually these cures are based on the assumption that conception is aided by relaxation, which there is little evidence to support. They might be advised that they can be sure that if they adopt they will instantly become pregnant. Or they might be told that they are trying too hard, to just relax, or to merely give the problem to God, or to make love as they always did and stop worrying about it. All of this good advice usually helps the man and his wife be even more anxious because they are not able to relax.

Finally, they might have tried various spiritual cures. They might negotiate with God, drawing on biblical accounts such as Hannah, who dedicated Samuel to God (1 Sam. 1:11). They might assume that their faith is insufficient, which might prompt them to increase their Bible reading and prayer time. They might repent of previous or current sins—especially sexual sins—and seek inner healing. They might even find their faith challenged and their beliefs about prayer, or God, or about the meaning of being an adopted child of

God threatened. They might abandon their faith in an unconscious attempt to manipulate God into giving them a child.

Throughout the second stage—defending the assumption of
fertility—the prominent issues are locus of control, responsibility, and uncertainty.[8] For many couples, the family may
be the only area of life in which they feel control. Infertility
treatment gives up control over the most private part of the
couple's relationship—their sexual relationship. Every detail of
their sexual encounters—frequency, duration, positions, postcoital behavior—is subjected to scrutiny and is modified under
the advice of an outsider.

As they face the increasing likelihood that one of them is
sterile, responsibility and blame must be faced. Families become involved. Parents and in-laws who want grandchildren
can be especially intrusive in the couple's lives.

All of the investigations are characterized by uncertainty.
The husband and wife are uncertain whether anything is
wrong, whether they are performing correctly, whether they
are wasting their time and money, whether anything will work.
They are uncertain over the potential changes in their work and
their relationship should they be found to be sterile, or not.
They are even uncertain whether they could accept an adopted
child, or whether they *could* adopt. People dislike uncertainty.
It is stressful and distressing.

Giving Up the Assumption

Sometimes the various cures "work" and conception occurs.
However, many times none of the cures works. For those
couples, the impact will often be enormous.[9] Often, medical
testing shows that the infertility is permanent. When the assumption of fertility dies, the husband and wife experience
numerous reactions.[10]

Surprise and shocked disbelief. As with most traumas, the
initial reaction is numbness and inability to grasp the implications of the finding. Emotions may or may not be expressed,
but usually there is a dreamlike, unreal quality to the person's
experience.

Sadness. Shock usually subsides within about twenty-four

hours and the reality of the permanence of infertility is felt. Despite their intentions to accept the doctor's findings philosophically, the husband and wife usually sense the news as loss and sadness; tears are usually close to the surface and are triggered by almost anything such as the sight of a child, or a book or television program that mentions children.

Sense of isolation. One can walk down most streets in the United States and see some woman who is conspicuously pregnant; however, one can almost never walk down a street and see someone who is conspicuously infertile. The lack of visibility and the secretness with which most people treat their infertility create a sense of isolation for the infertile couple. It often seems that no one understands and no one shares the experience. Because no one seems to understand, they might compound their isolation through social withdrawal.

Lowered self-esteem. Most people's sense of worth is partly built on the assumption that they will contribute to the future of humanity through producing offspring. When a man and woman find that they will be unable to fulfill that role, their sense of self-worth is diminished. Until they can find other ways to contribute to the future, they will continue to feel the loss of self-worth.

Confused self-image. The infertile person does not at first understand all the implications of his or her infertility. The person might think that sexuality is impaired through infertility, so his or her sexual identity is challenged. Such persons might also think that they have somehow been transformed into "infertile persons." They develop a tragic self-image. In their minds, an introduction to a stranger might be, "Hi, I'm _____ . I can't have children." The topic of infertility winds its way into most serious conversations. Although this is understandable at first because the trauma is present on such persons' minds, if they develop a long-lasting self-definition as infertile persons, they may have trouble coping with the difficulty.

Guilt. Even though they might have done nothing that directly caused the infertility, they often feel guilty, especially over past or present sexual sins. They might feel extreme guilt over premarital and extramarital sexual relationships, abortion (even if the husband is the one who has been determined to be infertile), homosexual experiences as a teenager, or other sexual experiences. They might feel that God is getting even or punishing them.

Anger. Anger and frustration are mingled and are often vented at a variety of objects. They might feel angry at abortion advocates, doctors, relatives, God, spouses, other couples who become pregnant, or people who abuse their children.

Grief. They have experienced a loss that is nonetheless real for being the loss of the potential to have children. However, because the loss is not visible, they can often deny the loss and fail to resolve it for long periods of time. The sadness and depression that are usually associated with grief are often present. Couples will often talk about their loss again and again, in what is called "obsessive social review," characteristic of any grief. Because there is social stigma associated with infertility, they may depend totally on their spouses to discuss the loss. Sometimes this can irritate the spouses because of the repetitive nature of the obsessive social review—like a broken record, again and again.

Of course, not every couple will be affected the same way. Stryker believes that some parts of a person's identity are more important than other parts. If a person defines his or her identity in terms of being a biological parent or progenitor, then that person will react more extremely to the loss of the assumption of fertility.[11]

In fact, motherhood is so important to large parts of our contemporary society—especially within profamily Christian circles—that women are usually the hardest hit, even if the husband is found to be infertile. Miall[12] observed that most wives who discover themselves to be infertile spontaneously label themselves as deviant and "failures," despite support from their spouses, families, and peers.

Accepting the Infertility

Grief usually ends when the grieving person makes a conscious decision to put the loss behind and decides how to live with the loss. Often this decision will encourage the infertile spouses to seek friends to talk with about how to manage their difficulties. The joy of sexual intercourse, often reduced during adjustment to the loss, can return and can even be enhanced as the man and woman are freed from the rigors of medical scrutiny and the pressures of having sexual intercourse solely for procreation.

People might cope with infertility in several ways. One couple I know has devoted much of its time to others. The man has been actively involved in coaching boys' sports—baseball and soccer—and the woman has been a civic leader, producing plays for the community. Both have acted in the plays and have been involved in the church choir as well as other church activities. Both, too, have been actively involved in making contributions to society through their careers. Despite having no children of their own, they have affected hundreds of adults and children throughout the community—to such an extent that they have received a community service award from their state governor. This is called role readjustment. One effect of assuming new and clearly defined roles is that they talk about infertility differently. Instead of treating infertility as something bad, requiring an "excuse," they merely give a "justification."[13] An excuse is an explanation in which one admits that a state of affairs is wrong but denies full responsibility for it. A justification is an explanation in which responsibility is accepted but the state of affairs is not perceived as necessarily bad.[14] The change in ways of accounting for the problem helps the person fully accept the infertility and loss of the role as parent.

Another option for coping with infertility is adoption. When a husband and wife decide to adopt, they do not give up the parent role. Yet they usually give up the role of *biological* parent. This is usually called "resolution" of infertility.[15] Before social caseworkers approve an infertile couple as potential adoptive parents, they usually want to see some evidence of resolution.[16]

Both Stigger[17] and Stout[18] describe the procedures for both agency and private adoption. There are several resources for learning more about adoption (see Appendix 6).

COUNSELING THE INFERTILE COUPLE

As with any counseling, the counselor should never try to intervene without understanding how persons are experiencing the problem.

Assessment

This includes an assessment of what the individual is feeling, what he or she is thinking (and thus what stage he or she is in), and what has been tried as ways to cope with the problem. Infertile couples often criticize others for their insensitivity and tendency to offer platitudes, unsolicited advice, and glib reassurances. The counselor must understand the experiences of the couple before attempting to help them adjust to their difficulties. Usually, assessment means listening carefully to how the individual spouses are handling their experiences and understanding exactly where they are and what they hope to get from the counselor.

Giving Help

The help you provide depends on the stage of the individuals in their infertility. Couples in the first stage of infertility—the assumption of infertility—will generally not seek the help of a counselor. Only when the problem begins to become evident might they seek advice. The counselor might be of help through providing referrals to physicians who do fertility testing or even through suggesting various home or spiritual cures for infertility.

In many cases, infertility is temporary. If the husband and wife have been trying to become pregnant for only a few months, the advice to relax might be sufficient to help them enjoy each other, though it will probably have no effect on whether or not they conceive. Sometimes God does discipline or correct his children by providing hardship, so it might also be appropriate for the counselor to suggest that they examine their lives for the presence of sin. Because many couples know this already, the counselor might only broach the topic. He or she will soon find whether the couple has already tried this. Often couples will be defensive about the suggestion that they have brought infertility on themselves through misbehavior, and this defensiveness can contaminate the future counseling relationship. My preference is rarely to mention this or to mention it only in passing, assuming that the man and woman have already examined themselves before God.

Stigger cautions that most couples who become upset with their counselors do so because counselors assume that infertility is due to sin or that infertility is merely a stimulus to pray, while the man and woman do not share those assumptions.[19] The counselor should advance his or her assumptions tentatively and then only after finding out what they think about the idea.

Those in the second stage of coping with infertility are likely to deny responsibility for the cause or cure of infertility. One way to accomplish this is by placing the responsibility on the counselor to explain the *cause* of the problem. Not being omniscient, counselors can rarely do this in a way that fully satisfies the couple and are well advised to explain the cause of infertility only tentatively.

Counselors will often not be sought in earnest until the husband and wife find they are permanently infertile. At that time, the counselor can help them with the full range of grief reactions and with blame within the marriage. They must be counseled that they are each other's best source of social support for coping with their difficulties.

Once they reach the fourth stage—acceptance of the infertility—they can be counseled in ways that will help them redirect their productive energy.

Information

The counselor can often be a rich source of information for them throughout the stages of infertility. The counselor can tell the couple about the stages of coping and prepare them for likely future stages. Understanding what is likely to happen and what others have experienced can help them accept their reactions as normal and help relieve the sense of isolation and withdrawal that they are likely to feel. Other helpful information includes the many reasons that are possible explanations for infertility. Although the counselor should avoid offering just one reason for the infertility, he or she might provide a catalogue of them for the couple to think about and examine to see how appropriate each is for them.

Finally, the counselor can help the couple understand the reactions of others to their infertility. Generally, people respond to infertility on the basis of their own experience. For example, someone who is experiencing difficulty in raising a child might be likely to react to the news that a couple is infertile by saying, "It's just as well. I wouldn't want to have to raise a child in this time."[20] People want to understand the experience of the infertile couple, but most of them project themselves into the situation and respond as if they were infertile rather than try to understand the other's experience. The counselor can help the husband and wife be more tolerant of the comments of others whom they consider rude or insensitive.

Skills

The counselor might be able to help the couple learn needed skills. For example, they might need to improve their communication skills or their ability to educate others sensitively and nonjudgmentally concerning their pain. The husband and wife who have come to accept their infertility might require assistance in replanning some of their marital and career goals.

Support

The counselor can usually provide the most support by simply listening to the couple and trying to understand their plight. In addition, he or she might help mobilize the couple's Christian community so that they can understand the couple's pain and support them in their decisions. Thoughtless remarks from people within the close community are often described as being among the most painful aspects of dealing with infertility.

PREVENTION

Although infertility cannot be prevented, many of the secondary problems associated with it can be prevented. For instance, insensitive remarks from people within the congregation can be lessened by educating them about ways to behave with an infertile couple. Stigger recommended six dos and don'ts for members of the community.[21]

1. Do start by asking. The man and woman are often isolated and ashamed of their infertility. Close friends can show their support by asking about whether they are having difficulty conceiving. Friends must resist the temptation to lighten the mood through humor, for humor is often misperceived by the couple.

2. Do listen. Friends should listen to the experience of the couple rather than project themselves into their experience. Try to show love by understanding them from their own perspective.

3. Don't offer unsolicited advice, cheap comfort, glib reassurance, or stories about someone who had it worse. These tactics do not generally provide relief but merely distance the friend from the experience of the couple.

4. Do offer support. Once friends have asked and listened, they can provide help such as referral to organizations that address the issue of infertility, e.g., The American Fertility Society, Resolve, or Stepping Stones Ministry:

The American Fertility Society
Administrative Office
1608 13th Avenue South, Suite 101
Birmingham, AL 35205
205–933–7222

Resolve, Inc.
P.O. Box 474
Belmont, MA 02178
617–484–2424

Stepping Stones Ministry
P.O. Box 11141
Wichita, KS 67211

Other support might direct the couple to books about fertility or to organizations and books about adoption (if they suggest that they might have an interest in adoption). For recommended readings about infertility and adoption, see Appendix 7.

5. Do stay in contact with the couple. They are tempted to withdraw from contact because of the isolation they feel. In

addition, some people are uncomfortable around couples they know to be infertile because they do not know how to help or are afraid that they might unwittingly offend them. It is important to keep in contact and try to maintain a normal relationship with them.

6. Don't be afraid to make a mistake. Most couples know when you care for them and are trying to love them. They will forgive the occasional mistake.

Another preventive measure is to provide a congregation with information about the extent of the problem of infertility and the impact of the problem on those who experience it. People within the congregation can then be more sensitive to others who are having difficulty conceiving. In addition, church leaders can oversee the activities of the church to insure that not all activities are oriented for families, providing couples a chance to have fellowship with each other without the presence of children.

Finally, couples who are infertile try to understand why infertility has happened to them. This inevitably involves them in wrestling with the problem of pain: Why do evil and pain exist? Either God is good but is not powerful enough to prevent evil and pain, or God is powerful enough to prevent evil and pain but is not good. The entire congregation can be educated about the many answers that have been provided for the problem of pain. This provides an inoculation against the difficulties when couples experience pain in their lives. As in the case of inoculation, the members of the congregation are introduced to the problem and are encouraged to build up their "antibodies" by considering the various arguments. Then, when a couple experiences pain, they can draw on their already existing defenses to help win the battle for their faith that is likely to ensue in times of adversity.

PART FOUR

CONCLUSION

CHAPTER ELEVEN

WHO'S IN CONTROL HERE?
A PERSONAL RESPONSE TO THIS BOOK

THIS IS THE FOURTH BOOK I HAVE WRITTEN,[1] and it has affected me more than any of the others. This book has forced me to wrestle repeatedly with emotional issues such as the death and handicaps of children, unplanned fertility, and unplanned infertility.

I have tried to use a varied writing style throughout the book so that you could experience with me the pain and tears of moving experiences as well as the humor necessary to cope with life. I have wanted you to be as emotionally involved with the book as I have been—to feel as well as to learn.

Much of my feeling has come from my own experiences with my family and with people whom I have known. We have

struggled with tough questions. The toughest one for me—
which this book has continually raised—is the problem of
pain. Over my last fifteen years as a Christian and counselor, I
have struggled regularly with why painful things happen.
I have heard and read many answers and debated the answers
with Christians and non-Christians. I have held several different views over time that were sufficient to satisfy me. Counselees, friends, and family have tested my beliefs. Just when I
have thought I had the penultimate understanding of God and
his purposes, my answers have been challenged. This book has
again shaken me loose from pat answers to life's basic questions, and initiated new growth.

I hope that you, too, have thought about the problem of pain
throughout this book, arriving at new insights through self-
examination or perhaps confirming the beliefs you began with.
Your counselees with problem pregnancies will certainly have
been thinking about the problem and experiencing it emotionally, and pat answers will rarely suffice for them.

The counseling room is not the debate lectern nor a pulpit,
although at rare times it resembles each. The counseling room
is for sharing the experience of a family, for rejoicing with
those who rejoice, for weeping with those who weep. There is
room for stating our values and beliefs to inform the family of
our position so they can make intelligent judgments about how
to interpret our counsel. But ultimately, the counseling room is
the place where the counselor has the opportunity to act as
prophet (speaking God's words to the counselee) and priest (in-
terceding with and for the counselee to God).

Counselees must wrestle with big questions such as the
meaning for them of a problem pregnancy, death, a malformed
child, or discovered permanent infertility. As their counselor,
we can help lead them but cannot make the journey for them.
Each person must arrive at an answer that satisfies him or her.

I believe that counselors can best help with this quest for
meaning if they are at peace about the big questions. Some
answer must satisfy us. However, I have been amazed for years
at how answers that satisfy me might not satisfy anyone else.

In the following pages, I have recorded some of my thinking about the problem of why painful things happen. I have

questioned and offered only a few of the possible answers. Although I doubt that anyone will agree with all that I have written, I hope my thoughts will provoke you to examine the issues afresh. I pray that you will be able to accept my thinking as something that works for me, without feeling that I am trying to persuade you to think in any particular way. I think your examination of these issues will make you a more sensitive and confident counselor.

A FEW POSSIBLE QUESTIONS AND ANSWERS ABOUT PAIN, SUFFERING, AND EVIL

Q: Rabbi Kushner tries to answer why bad things happen to good people. Why do bad things happen to good people?

One answer to Rabbi Kushner[2] is that there are no good people. All people are fallen. All are imperfect (Rom. 3:10; Ps. 14:1; Deut. 24:16). We are like giant mirrors with holes in them. Some mirrors are shattered; others simply have a few baseballs hit through them. None of the mirrors is perfect. Having all broken the law, we are all guilty of breaking the *whole* law (Gal. 3:10). It is like trying to phone God long distance. Whether we dial a number that is totally incorrect or one that is correct in all numbers except one, we will reach the wrong number. Even Paul said that there was nothing good within him (Rom. 7:18). A more intriguing and accurate question might be, why do *good* things happen to bad people? The answer would be because God loves us even though we don't deserve it. Grace.

But dismissing Rabbi Kushner's question by saying that we are not good people is not the whole story. People are created in God's image and are good (Gen. 1:27), but fallen (Rom. 5:14). Both good and bad coexist within us. We also live in a fallen world (Gen. 3:15) in which good and bad coexist. The heavenlies also involve both good and bad, though the good and bad exist in separate realms: Satan was banished from heaven (Isa. 14:12) and now rules as prince of the power of the air over earth (Eph. 2:2). Wherever we go, until Jesus comes again or until we exist with God, Jesus, and the Holy Spirit in paradise (Rev. 21:4), we see both good and evil, happiness and pain.

Q: How about the Christian? Isn't he or she good?

The Christian is redeemed and his or her sins are paid for. The Christian, too, has a new heart and spirit within (Ezek. 11:19; 36:26). They coexist with our spiritually dead, but sometimes still active, worldly spirit, which Paul calls the "flesh" (Rom. 7:23).

But even though the Christian is saved and redeemed and will ultimately be translated both physically and spiritually into perfect fellowship with God, the Christian is appointed to live his or her earthly life in a world that is fallen. Our salvation does not erase natural consequences that produce pain and suffering.

Q: Won't God prevent pain of those whom he loves?

In the heavenlies, good is separated from evil. In our fallen earth, good and evil are intermixed and are often inseparable. When people hold the belief that the Christian is insulated from evil, I believe that they are mistakenly hurrying God's ultimate plan. In his plan for us on earth, he has promised that we *will* suffer (Rom. 8:18; 1 Pet. 4:12, 13) and he has told us ways to handle the suffering. When the Bible talks of being pain-free and sin-free, I believe it is talking about our ultimate fate.

On earth, God does love us and care for us. He will prevent unnecessary suffering but not either necessary suffering or suffering that springs from the natural consequences of sin, except in rare occasions.

Q: Does God cause pain, suffering, and evil?

All events are multiply caused. For example, if I strike a tennis ball with my racket, it might soar into my opponent's court. What caused it to be propelled into my opponent's court? One cause is explainable by physics: the force applied to the ball at an angle of ten degrees from the horizontal with the ball attracted to the earth by the force of gravity gave it a trajectory that resulted in its striking the court.

A second cause is explainable by my intention. I wanted to strike the ball and direct it into my opponent's court. A more distant cause involves the decision to play tennis today. I decided to play my opponent and the final result of that cause was to direct a ball into his court. An even more distant cause was my decision to learn to play tennis, or God's decision to create me, or even to create the world. All events are caused by a multitude of proximal (near in time and space) causes and distal (far away in time and space) causes.

When many people ask what *causes* suffering, they assume that there is only *one* cause. Either "the world" or God or Satan causes suffering. But the physics of pain, the psychology of pain, and the spirituality of pain are simply different levels of causality. Being able to explain physically or chromosomally how a baby became handicapped does not negate the psychological explanation nor the spiritual explanation.

We know from Scripture that God does not cause *evil*. God is separate from evil and it is against his character. Evil exists only because God has not yet ended it (which he will some day), but God does not *cause* evil.

Nonetheless, God allows Satan to cause evil (see Job) because God uses the evil to accomplish his ultimate purposes, and "in everything God works for good with those who love him, who are called according to his purpose" (Rom. 8:28). God is our heavenly Father who gives us everything we need, not our heavenly grandfather who gives us everything we want.

Q: How does God work within painful circumstances?

First, we must recognize that "painful circumstances" is a limiting way of thinking about pain. Life moves onward continuously and God can act differently from minute to minute. To help understand this, take a simplified account of pain. We might think of it in four stages:

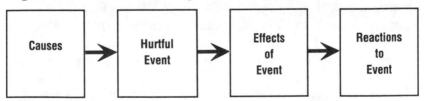

The *causes* of the hurtful event may be traced distally to the Fall and to God's curses that came about as a consequence of the sin of Adam and Eve (Gen. 3:15). Or the causes may be as proximal as God supernaturally intervening as a punishment for habitual sin (Heb. 12:5). Or God may be at work in the life of a person so that he allows the person to sin in hopes that he or she will ultimately repent (Rom. 1:24, 26; 1 Cor. 5:5). Unfortunately, that sin might ultimately result in a *hurtful event* in the life of the Christian. God may be at work on many levels of causality.

Further, God may be at work in the *effects* of the hurtful event. He has been at work distally in that he created natural law, the law of cause and effect, when he created the earth. He may be at work more proximally by supernaturally protecting someone (because of the prayers of the believer [Ps. 41:2]) from what ordinarily would have been natural consequences.

Further, God may be at work in the *reactions* people have to hurtful events. He is at work distally in that he has allowed other Christians to suffer and be comforted so they can provide comfort to the person suffering in this event (2 Cor. 1:3–4). He may be at work more proximally through the Holy Spirit's conviction of the person over his or her bitter reaction to the hurtful event.

God is at work throughout painful circumstances on all levels to accomplish his purposes. These actions do not necessarily conflict with other causes. God often works through natural physical causes and sometimes he intervenes supernaturally. Sometimes his will and the will of others conflict and that does not always mean that the other person will not get his or her way. In the case of Joseph, his brothers meant his sale into slavery for evil, but God meant it for good (Gen. 50:20).

Q: How about our responsibility in painful circumstances?

We are responsible for obeying God and for seeking his will in all aspects of painful circumstances. We are to pursue God's character and his will in the causes of events, in the effects of the events, and in our reactions to the events. God's way is always to seek closer contact with him, though how that is accomplished in each case is not always clear.

Q: If Christians are sincerely trying to seek God's will and God works in everything for good, how can we still experience pain?

God is not overly concerned with the happiness of the believer at all times. Surprisingly, he is not always concerned about the faith of the believer. More important to God is the *character* of the believer. Faith is appropriate only when we walk the earth. When we see God face to face, faith will be unnecessary (1 Cor. 13:2, 10; 2 Cor. 1:3, 4). All that will matter then is how we love God and what our character is. God desires our eternal joy in harmonious fellowship and love with him. He sometimes uses our temporal pain to accomplish growth in our character and in our love and trust of him. God is good. There are many reasons that he allows pain:

a. To build faith. Although faith is of little eternal significance (since it will pass away), it is of great temporal importance. God wants us to choose faith at every point in painful circumstances—in causes, effects, and reactions to painful events.

b. To permit a demonstration of his power. Jesus explained to the blind man at the temple that he had been born blind not because of his or anyone's sin but so that God's works could be made manifest through him (John 9:3).

c. To build our character. "More than that, we rejoice in our sufferings, knowing that suffering produces endurance, and endurance produces character . . . " (Rom. 5:3, 4a).

d. To correct us. ". . . says the Lord. In vain have I smitten your children, they took no correction" (Jer. 2:30a; see also Jer. 5:3).

e. To discipline us. "For the Lord disciplines him whom he loves. . . . It is for discipline that you have to endure. . . . For the moment all discipline seems painful rather than pleasant; later it yields the peaceful fruit of righteousness to those who have been trained by it" (Heb. 12:6a, 7a, 11).

f. To get our attention. C. S. Lewis described pain as "God's megaphone to rouse the ear of a deaf world."[3]

g. To train us to comfort others. "Blessed be the God and Father of our Lord Jesus Christ, the Father of mercies and God of all comfort, who comforts us in all our affliction, so that we may be able to comfort those who are in any affliction, with the comfort with which we ourselves are comforted by God" (2 Cor. 1:3, 4).

Q: How can we handle suffering?

We are told to "rejoice in our suffering" (Rom. 5:3). This does not say "don't suffer." We are not to pretend that pain is not painful or that illness is not illness. But we are to look to

God for our salvation and for our help. We are to trust him as good. We are to experience the challenges to our faith that pain brings and recall the mercies of the Lord, finally moving beyond the suffering to trust and strength of character instead of mistrust, unbelief, and bitterness.

Q: What am I to do as a counselor of those in pain?

First, I am not called to take away the pain from such persons. Nor am I called to provide meaning or understanding for them. I am called to be with them and to offer them the comfort of my presence, which is the comfort that God offers me in my affliction (2 Cor. 1:3, 4). At times this might entail giving helpful advice, information (see Appendix 8 for recommended readings), or even giving confrontation when I am sure that the counselee needs it. Mostly, it involves giving human compassion and love as one member in the body of Christ. As a counselor of families with problem pregnancies, I do not need to have all the answers. I should prepare myself responsibly for what God has called me to do, but he is the one who is the Savior of the lost, troubled, and distressed. Who's in control here? The triune God.

APPENDIX 1

RECOMMENDED READINGS CONCERNING ADOLESCENT PREGNANCY

For the Counselor About Adolescence and Pregnancy

Burtchaell, James T. *Rachel Weeping: The Case Against Abortion* (San Francisco: Harper and Row, 1982).

Delahoyde, Melinda. *Fighting for Life: Defending the Newborn's Right to Live* (Ann Arbor, Mich.: Servant Books, 1984).

Elkind, David. "Egocentrism in Adolescence," *Child Development* 38 (1967): 1025–64.

Fisher, Roger, and Ury, William. *Getting to Yes: Negotiating Agreement Without Giving In* (New York: Penguin Books, 1981).

Jorgensen, Stephen R., and Sonstegard, Janet S. "Predicting Adolescent Sexual and Contraceptive Behavior: An Application and Test of the Fishbein Model," *Journal of Marriage and the Family* 46 (1984): 43–55.

Kazdin, Alan E. (ed). "Special Issue: Psychotherapy Research," *Journal of Consulting and Clinical Psychology* 54 (1986): 3–117.

Marshner, C. "Once Conceived, A Child Has the Right to Be Born," in Feldman, Harold and Margaret. *Current Controversies in Marriage and Family* (Beverly Hills, Calif.: Sage, 1985), pp. 203–11.

Reagan, Ronald. "Abortion and the Conscience of the Nation," *Human Life Review* (Spring, 1983).

Schaeffer, Francis, and Koop, C. Everett. *What Ever Happened to the Human Race?* (Old Tappan, N.J.: Fleming H. Revell, 1979).

Young, Curt. *The Least of These: What Everyone Should Know About Abortion* (Chicago: Moody Press, 1983).

For the Pregnant Adolescent About the Decisions She Must Make

Allen, R. *What's the Matter with Christy?* (Minneapolis: Bethany House, 1982).

O'Brien, B. *Mom . . . I'm Pregnant* (Wheaton, Ill.: Tyndale House, 1982).

Owens, C., and Roggow, L. *Handbook for Pregnant Teenagers* (Minneapolis: Bethany House, 1984).

Walling, R. *When Pregnancy Is a Problem?* (St. Meinrad, Ind.: Abbey Press, 1980).

For the Adolescent Mother About Parenting

Azrin, Nathan H., and Fox, Richard M. *Toilet Training in Less Than a Day* (New York: Pocket Books, 1974).

Beck, J. *How to Raise a Brighter Child* (New York: Pocket Books, 1967).

Becker, W. *Parents Are Teachers: A Child Management Program,* (Champaign, Ill.: Research Press 1971).

Dobson, J. *Dare to Discipline* (Wheaton, Ill.: Tyndale House, 1970).

Kesler, J. *Family Forum* (Wheaton, Ill.: Victor Books, 1984).

Leman, K. *Making Children Mind Without Losing Yours* (Old Tappan, N.J.: Fleming H. Revell, 1984).

Narramore, B. *Help! I'm a Parent* (Grand Rapids, Mich.: Zondervan, 1972).

Owen, P. H. *Seven Styles of Parenting* (Wheaton, Ill.: Tyndale House, 1983).

Richards, L. O. *The Word Parents Handbook* (Waco, Tex.: Word, 1983).

Schaeffer, E. *The Hidden Art of Homemaking* (Wheaton, Ill.: Tyndale House, 1985).

Sears, W. *Christian Parenting and Child Care* (Nashville: Thomas Nelson, 1985).

For the Adolescent and Her Family About Adoption

Burgess, L.C. *The Art of Adoption* (New York: Norton, 1981).

Lindsay, J. W. *Pregnant Too Soon: Adoption Is an Option* (St. Paul, Minn.: EMC Publishing, 1980).

Owens, C., and Roggow, L. *Handbook for Pregnant Teenagers* (Grand Rapids, Mich.: Zondervan, 1984).

Zimmerman, M. *Should I Keep My Baby?* (Minneapolis: Bethany House, 1983).

APPENDIX 2

RECOMMENDED READINGS CONCERNING COHABITATION

Berger, B., and P. L. *The War Over the Family: Capturing the Middle Ground* (Garden City, N.Y.: Anchor Press/Doubleday, 1984).

Clark, K. *An Experience of Chastity: A Creative Reflection on Intimacy, Loneliness, Sexuality, and Commitment* (Notre Dame, Ind.: Ave Maria Press, 1982).

Inmon, M.N., and Wright, H.N. *Preparing for Parenthood* (Ventura, Calif.: Regal Books, 1980).

Leman, K. *Smart Girls Don't: And Guys Don't Either* (Ventura, Calif.: Regal Books, 1982).

Schaeffer, F. *A Time for Anger: The Myth of Neutrality* (Westchester, Ill.: Crossway Books, 1982).

White, J. *Eros Defiled: The Christian and Sexual Sin* (Downers Grove, Ill.: InterVarsity Press, 1977).

APPENDIX 3

RECOMMENDED READINGS FOR PREPARING FOR A BABY

Bacher, J. M. *A Mother's Joy* (Grand Rapids, Mich.: Baker, 1983).

Coleman, W. L. *Getting Ready for Our New Baby* (Minneapolis: Bethany House, 1984).

Davity, L. L. *Baby Hunger: Every Woman's Longing for a Baby* (Minneapolis: Winston Press, 1984).

Eagen, A. B. *The Newborn Mother: Stages of Her Growth* (New York: Little, Brown, 1985).

Inmon, M. N., and Wright, H.N. *Preparing for Parenthood* (Ventura, Calif.: Regal Books, 1980).

Walter, C. A. *The Timing of Motherhood* (Lexington, Mass.: Lexington Books, 1986).

APPENDIX 4

RECOMMENDED READINGS FOR PARENTING CHILDREN WITH SPECIAL DIFFICULTIES

Difficult Children

Kirkland, J. "Infant Crying—Problem That Won't Go Away!" *Parents' Centre Bulletin* 96 (1983): 15–17.

Kirkland, J., Deane, F., and Brennan, M. "About CrySOS, A Clinic for People with Crying Babies," *Family Relations* 32 (1983): 537–43.

LaRossa, R. *Becoming a Parent* (Beverly Hills, Calif.: Sage, 1986).

Mentally Retarded Children

Apgar, V., and Beck, J. *Is My Baby All Right?* (New York: Trident Press, 1973).

Rogers, D. *Angel Unaware* (Old Tappan, N.J.: Fleming H. Revell, 1956).

Physical Handicaps

Apgar, V., and Beck, J. *Is My Baby All Right?* (New York: Trident Press, 1973).

Klaus, M.H., and Kennell, J. H. *Maternal-Infant Bonding: The Impact of Early Separation or Loss on Family Development* (St. Louis: Mosby, 1976).

Chronic Illness

See Patterson and McCubbin, "Chronic Illness: Family Stress and Coping," for a summary of the different tasks of the family throughout the life cycle of the handicapped or chronically ill child.

McCubbin, H. I., McCubbin, M., Patterson, J. M., Cauble, A., Wilson, L., and Warwick, W. "CHIP—Coping Health Inventory for Parents: An Assessment of Parental Coping Patterns in the Case of the Chronically Ill Child," *Journal of Marriage and the Family* (1984).

Travis, G. *Chronic Illness in Children* (Stanford: Stanford University Press, 1976).

APPENDIX 5

RECOMMENDED READINGS ABOUT PROBLEMS ASSOCIATED WITH BIRTH TO MIDLIFE PARENTS

Midlife Crisis

Conway, J. *Men in Midlife Crisis* (Elgin, Ill.: David C. Cook Publishing, 1978).

Babies After 30

Berezin, N. *After a Loss in Pregnancy: Help for Families Affected by a Miscarriage, a Stillbirth, or the Loss of a Newborn* (New York: Simon and Schuster, 1982).

Bing, E., and Coleman, L. *Having a Baby After 30: Reassurance and Professional Guidance for Couples Who Waited* (New York: Bantam Books, 1980).

Cohen, J. B. *Parenthood After 30? A Guide to Personal Choice* (Lexington, Mass.: Lexington Books, 1985).

Daniels, P., and Weingarten, K. *Sooner or Later: The Timing of Parenthood* (New York: Norton, 1982).

Kappelman, M. M., and Ackerman, P. R. *Parents After Thirty* (New York: Rawson, Wade, 1980).

High-Risk Pregnancy

Freeman, R., and Pescar, P. *Safe Delivery: Protecting Your Baby During High-Risk Pregnancy* (New York: McGraw-Hill, 1983).

Hales, D., and Creasy, R. K. *New Hope for Problem Pregnancies* (New York: Harper and Row, 1982).

Infant Death

Borg, S., and Lasker, J. *When Pregnancy Fails: Families Coping with Miscarriage, Stillbirth, and Infant Death* (Boston: Beacon Press, 1981).

DeFrain, J., Martens, L., Stork, J., and Stork, W. *Stillborn: The Invisible Death* (Lexington, Mass.: Lexington Books, 1986).

Grollman, E. (ed). *Explaining Death to Children* (Boston: Beacon Press, 1979).

Pizer, H., and Palinski, C. O. *Coping with a Miscarriage* (New York: The Dial Press, 1982).

APPENDIX 6

RESOURCES FOR INFORMATION ABOUT ADOPTION

Bethany Christian Services
Central Office
901 Eastern, N.E.
Grand Rapids, MI 49503
616–459–6273

National Committee for Adoption
1346 Connecticut Avenue, N.W., Suite 326
Washington, D.C. 20036
National Adoption Hotline: 202 463–7563

North American Center for Adoption
67 Irving Place
New York, NY 10003
212–254–7410

Organizations specializing in adoptions of foreign children

Holt Adoption Program
P.O. Box 2420
Eugene, OR 97402

International Social Services
291 Broadway
New York, NY 10007

Los Ninos International
1106 Random Circle
Austin, TX 78745

OURS (Organization for a United Response)
3307 Highway 100 North, Suite 203
Minneapolis, MN 55422

World Family Adoptions, Inc.
5048 Fairy Chasu Road
West Bend, WI 43095

For organizations specializing in adoption of needy children or hard to place children:

AASK (Aid to Adoption of Special Kids)
3530 Grand Avenue
Oakland, CA 94610

The Adoption Center of Delaware Valley
1218 Chestnut Street
Philadelphia, PA 19107

CAP Book
700 Exchange Street
Rochester, NY 14608

North American Council on Adoptable Children
1346 Connecticut Avenue, N.W.
Washington, D.C. 20036

APPENDIX 7

RECOMMENDED READINGS ABOUT INFERTILITY AND ADOPTION

Infertility

Decker, A., and Zoebl, S. *Why Can't We Have a Baby?* (New York: Warner Books, 1979).

Eck-Menning, B. *Infertility: A Guide for the Childless Couple* (Englewood Cliffs, N.J.: Prentice-Hall, 1977).

Silber, S. J. *How to Get Pregnant* (New York: Charles Scribner and Sons, 1980).

Stangel, J. J. *Fertility and Conception: An Essential Guide for Childless Couples* (New York: Paddington Press, Ltd., 1979).

Stigger, J. A. *Coping With Infertility: A Guide for Couples, Families, and Counselors* (Minneapolis: Augsburg, 1983).

Stout, M. *Without Child: A Compassionate Look at Infertility* (Grand Rapids, Mich.: Zondervan, 1985).

Adoption

Burgess, Linda C. *The Art of Adoption* (New York: W. W. Norton, 1981).

Carney, A. *Nor More Here and There: Adopting the Older Child* (Chapel Hill, N.C.: University of North Carolina Press, 1976).

Dywasuk, C. *Adoption—Is It for You?* (New York: Harper and Row, 1973).

Gilman, L. *The Adoption Resource Book* (New York: Harper and Row, 1984).

Jewett, C. *Adopting the Older Child* (Boston: Harvard Common Press, 1977).

Kravik, P. J. *Adopting Children with Special Needs* (New York: North American Council on Adoptable Children, 1976).

Krementz, J. *How It Feels To Be Adopted* (New York: Alfred A. Knopf, 1982).

Martin, C.D. *Beating the Adoption Game* (San Diego: Oak Tree, 1980).

McNamara, J. *The Adoption Adviser* (New York: Hawthorne Books, 1975).

Plumez, J. H. *Successful Adoption: A Guide to Finding a Child and Raising a Family* (New York: Crown Publishers, 1982).

Raymond, L. *Adoption and After* (New York: Harper and Row, 1974).

Shireman, J. F., and Johnson, P. R. *Adoption: Three Alternatives—A Comparative Study of Three Alternative Forms of Adoptive Placement, Phase II* (Chicago: Chicago Child Care Society, 1980).

Sorosky, A. D., Baron, A., and Pannor, R. *The Adoption Triangle* (New York: Anchor Press/Doubleday, 1978).

Stein, L. M., and Hoopers, J. L. *Identity Formation in the Adopted Adolescent* (New York: Child Welfare League of America, 1985).

VanWhy, E. W. *Adoption Bibliography and Multi-Ethnic Sourcebook* (Hartford, Conn.: Open Door Society of Connecticut, 1977).

APPENDIX 8

RECOMMENDED READINGS ABOUT
THE PROBLEM OF PAIN

Baker, D. *Pain's Hidden Purpose: Finding Perspective in the Midst of Suffering* (Portland, Ore.: Multnomah Press, 1984).

Landorf, J. *The High Cost of Growing* (New York: Bantam, 1979).

Lewis, C. S. *A Grief Observed* (New York: Seabury Press, 1961).

Lewis, C. S. *The Problem of Pain* (New York: Macmillan, 1962).

Ogilvie, L. J. *If God Cares, Why Do I Still Have Problems?* (Waco, Tex.: Word, 1985).

Schaeffer, E. *Affliction* (Old Tappan, N.J.: Fleming H. Revell, 1978).

Yancey, P. *Where Is God When It Hurts?* (Grand Rapids, Mich.: Zondervan, 1977).

NOTES

Introduction

1. Everett L. Worthington, Jr., "Religious Counseling: A Review of Published Empirical Research," *Journal of Counseling and Development* 64 (1986): 421–31.

Chapter 1 An Overview of Unplanned Pregnancies

1. I am indebted to Jim Goalder for this story.
2. A. Browne and D. Finkelhor, "Impact of Child Sexual Abuse," *Psychological Bulletin* 99 (1986): 66–71; R. I. Lanyon, "Theory and Treatment in Child Molestation," *Journal of Consulting and Clinical Psychology* 54 (1986): 176–182; Lizette Peterson and L. Mori, "Prevention of Child Injury: An Overview of Targets, Methods, and Tactics for Psychologists," *Journal of Consulting and Clinical Psychology* 53 (1986): 586–95; J. E. Rolf, "Evolving Adaptive Theories and Methods for Prevention Research with Children," *Journal of Consulting and Clinical Psychology* 53 (1985): 631–46; M. S. Rosenberg and N. D. Repucci, "Primary Prevention of Child Abuse," *Journal of Consulting and Clinical Psychology* 53 (1985): 576–85.
3. Select Committee on Children, Youth, and Families, U.S. House of Representatives, *Teen Pregnancy: What Is Being Done?* A

State-by-State Look—Minority Views (Washington, D.C.: U.S. Government Printing Office, 1986).

4. P. Lewis, *40 Ways to Teach Your Child Values* (Wheaton, Ill.: Tyndale House, 1985).

5. Carol Anderson, "Community Connection: The Impact of Social Networks on Family and Individual Functioning," in Fromma Walsh (ed), *Normal Family Processes* (New York: Guilford, 1982), 425–45.

6. Tim LaHaye, *The Battle for the Family* (Old Tappan, N.J.: Fleming H. Revell, 1982).

Chapter 2 Crisis and Life Transition

1. Alice S. Rossi, "Transition to Parenthood," *Journal of Marriage and the Family* 30 (1968): 26, 39.

2. Reuben Hill, *Families Under Stress* (New York: Harper and Row, 1949).

3. Hamilton I. McCubbin and Joan M. Patterson, "Family Stress and Adaptation to Crisis: A Double ABCX Model of Family Behavior," in David H. Olson and Brent Miller, eds., *Family Studies Review Yearbook* (Beverly Hills, Calif.: Sage Publications, 1983).

4. David H. Olson, Hamilton I. McCubbin, H. Barnes, A. Larsen, M. Muxen, and M. Wilson, *Families: What Makes Them Work* (Beverly Hills, Calif.: Sage Publications, 1983); see also J. A. Petersen, *Conquering Family Stress* (Wheaton, Ill.: Victor Books, 1978) and James Dobson, *Love Must Be Tough: New Hope for Families in Crisis* (Waco, Tex.: Word, 1983).

5. Olson, McCubbin *et al.*, *Families.*

6. Evelyn Duvall, *Marriage and Family Development, 5th ed.* (New York: J.P. Lippincott, 1977).

7. Gail Sheehy, *Passages: Predictable Crises of Adult Life* (Toronto: Bantam Books, 1976).

8. Steven J. Danish, M. A. Smyer, and C. A. Nowak, "Developmental Intervention: Enhancing Life-event Processes," in Paul B. Baltes and Orville G. Brim, Jr., eds., *Life Span Development and Behavior,* vol. 3 (New York: Academic Press, 1980).

9. Bill Cosby, *Fatherhood* (Garden City, N.Y.: Doubleday, 1986).

10. Worthington, and Beverley G. Buston, "The Marriage Relationship in the Transition to Parenthood: A Review and a Model," *Journal of Family Issues* 9 (1987): 109–19.

11. Norval D. Glenn and Sara McLanahan, "Children and Marital Happiness: A Further Specification of the Relationship," *Journal of Marriage and the Family* 44 (1982): 63–72; Norval D. Glenn and Charles N. Weaver, "A Multivariate, Multisurvey Study of Marital Happiness," *Journal of Marriage and the Family* 40 (1978): 269–82; Linda C. Harriman, "Personal and Marital Changes Accompanying Parenthood," *Family Relations* 32 (1983): 387–94; Ralph LaRossa, "The Transition to Parenthood and the Social Reality of Time," *Journal of Marriage and the Family* 45 (1983): 579–89; Margaret M. Marini, *Consequences of Childbearing and Childspacing Patterns for Parents,* final report submitted to NICHD under Contract No. 1-HD-52840, Battelle Human Affairs Research Centers, Seattle, Wash.; Brent C. Miller, "A Multivariate Developmental Model of Marital Satisfaction," *Journal of Marriage and the Family* 38 (1976): 643–57; Judith A. Myers-Walls, "Balancing Multiple Role Responsibilities During the Transition to Parenthood," *Family Relations* 33 (1984): 267–71; Susan R. Orden and Norman M. Bradburn, "Dimensions of Marriage Happiness," *American Journal of Sociology* 73 (1968): 715–31; Douglas K. Snyder, "Multidimensional Assessment of Marital Satisfaction," *Journal of Marriage and the Family* 41 (1979): 812–23.

12. James F. Alexander and Bruce V. Parsons, *Functional Family Therapy* (Monterey, Calif.: Brooks/Cole, 1973); Coles Barton and James F. Alexander, "Functional Family Therapy," in Alan T. Gurman and David P. Kniskern, eds., *Handbook of Family Therapy* (New York: Brunner/Mazel, 1981), 403–43.

13. Michael Argyle and Adrian Furnham, "Sources of Satisfaction and Conflict in Long-term Relationships," *Journal of Marriage and the Family* 45 (1983): 795–803; N. Jacobson, H. Waldron, and D. Moore, "Toward a Behavioral Profile of Marital Distress," *Journal of Consulting and Clinical Psychology* 48 (1980): 696–703.

14. Jay Haley, *Strategies of Psychotherapy* (New York: Grune and Stratton, 1963).

15. Haley, *Strategies of Psychotherapy;* Carlos E. Sluzki, "Marital Therapy from a Systems Theory Perspective," in Thomas J. Paolino and Barbara S. McCrady, eds., *Marriage and Marital Therapy* (New York: Brunner/Mazel, 1978), 366–94; Paul Watzlawick, Janet B. Bavelas, and Don Jackson, *Pragmatics of Human Communication* (New York: Norton, 1967).

16. David H. Olson, Candyce S. Russell, and Douglas H. Sprenkle, "Circumplex Model VI: Theoretical Update," *Family Processes* 22 (1983): 69–83.

17. Jay Belsky and Michael Rovine, "Social-network Contact, Family Support, and the Transition to Parenthood," *Journal of Marriage and the Family* 46 (1984): 455–62; J. Belsky, G. Spanier, and M. Rovine, "Stability and Change in Marriage Across the Transition to Parenthood," *Journal of Marriage and the Family* 45 (1983): 567–77; Myers-Walls, "Balancing Multiple Role Responsibilities During the Transition to Parenthood."

Chapter 3 Counseling Families During Transitions

1. Donald J. Kiesler, "Some Myths of Psychotherapy Research and the Search for a Paradigm," *Psychological Bulletin* 65 (1966): 110–36.
2. Alan E. Kazdin (ed), "Special Issue: Psychotherapy Research," *Journal of Consulting and Clinical Psychology* 54 (1986): 3–117; Hans J. Strupp, S. W. Hadley, and B. Gomez-Schwartz, *Psychotherapy for Better or Worse* (New York: Jason Aronson, 1977); Gary R. VandenBos, ed., "Special Issue: Psychotherapy Research," *American Psychologist* 41 (1986): 111–214.
3. Kazdin, "Special Issue," 3.
4. Worthington, *When Someone Asks for Help: A Practical Manual for Counseling* (Downers Grove, Ill.: InterVarsity Press, 1982).
5. Worthington, "Religious Counseling."
6. Jay Haley, *Problem Solving Therapy* (San Francisco: Jossey-Bass, 1976).
7. Haley, *Problem Solving Therapy.*
8. Salvador Minuchin and H. Charles Fishman, *Family Therapy Techniques* (Cambridge, Mass.: Harvard University Press, 1981).
9. Gerald R. Patterson, *Coercive Family Process: A Social Learning Approach* (Eugene, Ore.: Castalia Publishing Co., 1982).
10. Worthington, *When Someone Asks for Help.*
11. Roger Fisher and William Ury, *Getting to Yes: Negotiating Agreement Without Giving In* (New York: Penguin Books, 1981).

Chapter 4 Teenage Pregnancy

1. Alan Guttmacher Institute, *11 Million Teenagers* (New York: Planned Parenthood Federation of America, 1976).
2. Select Committee on Children, Youth, and Families, U.S. House of Representatives, *Teen Pregnancy—Minority Views*.

3. Jean Piaget and B. Inhelder, *The Psychology of the Child* (New York: Basic Books, 1969).

4. Margaret Donaldson, "The Mismatch Between School and Children's Minds," *Human Nature* (1979): 60–7.

5. David Elkind, "Egocentricism in Adolescence," *Child Development* 38 (1967): 1025–34.

6. Lawrence Kohlberg, "Revisions in the Theory and Practice of Moral Development," *New Directions for Child Development* 2 (1978): 83–8.

7. J. R. Snarey, "Cross-cultural Universality of Social-Moral Development: A Critical Review of Kohlbergian Research," *Psychological Bulletin* 97 (1985): 202–32.

8. J. Lewis, *How's Your Family?* (New York: Brunner/Mazel, 1979).

9. Erik H. Erikson, *Identity, Youth and Crisis* (New York: Norton, 1968).

10. H. D. Thornburg, "The Amount of Sex Information Learning Obtained During Early Adolescence," *Journal of Early Adolescence* 1 (1981): 171–83.

11. Cynthia A. Clark and Everett L. Worthington, Jr., "Family Variables Affecting the Transmission of Religious Values from Parents to Adolescents: A Review," *Family Perspective* 21 (1987): 1–21.

12. Lawrence Steinberg and John P. Hill, "Patterns of Family Interaction as a Function of Age, the Onset of Puberty, and Formal Thinking," *Developmental Psychology* 14 (1978): 683–84.

13. John P. Hill, Grayson N. Holmbeck, Lynn Marlow, T. M. Green, and M. E. Lynch, "Menarcheal Status and Parent-Child Relations in Families of Seventh-Grade Girls," *Journal of Youth and Adolescence* 14 (1985): 301–16.

14. R. Pannor, F. Massarik, and B. Evans, *The Unwed Father: New Approaches for Helping Unmarried Young Parents* (New York: Springer, 1971).

15. V. Abernathy, "Illegitimate Conception Among Teenagers," *American Journal of Public Health* 64 (1974): 662–65.

16. N. Perry and C. R. Millemit, "Child Rearing Antecedents of Low and High Anxiety Eighth-Grade Children," in Charles D. Spielberger and Ira G. Sarason, eds., *Stress and Anxiety* (Washington, D.C.: Hemisphere, 1977).

17. J. D. Paulker, "Girls Pregnant Out of Wedlock," *Journal of Operational Psychology* 1 (1970): 7; H. B. Kaplan, P. B. Smith, and A. D. Pokorny, "Psychosocial Antecedents of Unwed Motherhood

Among Indigent Adolescents," *Journal of Youth and Adolescence* 8 (1979): 181–207.

18. J. Cheetham, *Unplanned Pregnancy and Counseling* (London: Routedge and Kegan Paul, 1977).

19. Joseph H. Meyerowitz and J. S. Maler, "Pubescent Attitudinal Correlates Antecedent to Adolescent Illegitimate Pregnancy," *Journal of Youth and Adolescence* 2 (1973): 251–8.

20. S. Fisher and K. R. Scharf, "Teenage Pregnancy: An Anthropological, Sociological, and Psychological Overview," *Adolescent Psychiatry* 8 (1980): 393–403.

21. Jay Haley, *Leaving Home: A Therapy of Disturbed Young People* (New York: McGraw-Hill, 1981).

22. A.S. Friedman, *Therapy with Families of Sexually Acting Out Girls* (New York: Springer, 1971); L. Klein, "Antecedents to Teenage Pregnancy," *Clinical Obstetrics and Gynecology* 32 (1978): 1151–59.

23. H. Stierlin, *Separating Parents and Adolescents: A Perspective on Running Away, Schizophrenia, and Waywardness* (New York: Quadrangle, 1974).

24. C. Vincent, *Unmarried Mothers* (New York: Free Press of Glencoe, 1961).

25. Group for the Advancement of Psychiatry, *Crises of Adolescence. Teenage Pregnancy: Impact on Adolescent Development* (New York: Brunner/Mazel, 1986).

26. Pannor *et al.*, *The Unwed Father.*

27. Frank Furstenberg, *Unplanned Parenthood: The Social Consequences of Teenage Childbearing* (New York: Free Press, 1976).

28. P. Rains, *Becoming an Unwed Mother* (Chicago and New York: Aldine/Atherton, 1971).

29. Elkind, "Egocentricism in Adolescence."

30. R. H. Rosen, "Adolescent Pregnancy Decision-Making: Are Parents Important?" *Adolescence* 15 (1980).

31. J. D. Osofsky and H. J. Osofsky, "Teenage Pregnancy: Psychosocial Considerations," *Clinical Obstetrics and Gynecology* 21:4 (1978): 1161–73.

32. C. E. Bowerman, D. P. Irish, and H. Pope, *Unwed Motherhood—Personal and Social Consequences* (Chapel Hill: University of North Carolina Institute for Research in the Social Sciences, 1963–66, 1966); E. H. Pohlman, *The Psychology of Birth Planning* (Cambridge, Mass.: Schenkman Press, 1969).

33. Bowerman *et al.*, *Unwed Motherhood.*

34. R. Bernstein, *Helping Unmarried Mothers* (New York: Association Press, 1971).

35. H. J. Osofsky, J. W. Hagen, and P. W. Wood, "A Program for Pregnant School Girls—Some Early Results," *American Journal of Obstetrics and Gynecology* 100 (1968): 1020.

36. Mark W. Roosa, H. E. Fitzgerald, and N. A. Carlson, "A Comparison of Teenage and Older Mothers: A Systems Analysis," *Journal of Marriage and the Family* 44 (1982): 367–77.

37. Select Committee on Children, Youth, and Families, U.S. House of Representatives, *Teen Pregnancy—Minority Views.*

38. Roosa *et al.*, "A Comparison of Teenage and Older Mothers."

39. Rains, *Becoming an Unwed Mother.*

40. Bowerman *et al.*, *Unwed Motherhood.*

41. Roosa *et al.*, "A Comparison of Teenage and Older Mothers," 15.

42. Furstenberg, *Unplanned Parenthood.*

43. Frank G. Bolton, Jr., *The Pregnant Adolescent: Problems of Premature Parenthood* (Beverly Hills, Calif.: Sage, 1980).

44. Furstenberg, *Unplanned Parenthood.*

45. Bolton, *The Pregnant Adolescent.*

46. George Ainslie, "Specious Reward: A Behavioral Theory of Impulsiveness and Impulse Control," *Psychological Bulletin* 82 (1975): 463–96.

47. Icek Ajzen and Martin Fishbein, *Understanding Attitudes and Predicting Social Behavior* (Englewood Cliffs, N.J.: Prentice-Hall, 1980).

48. Stephen R. Jorgensen and Janet S. Sonstegard, "Predicting Adolescent Sexual and Contraceptive Behavior: An Application and Test of the Fishbein Model," *Journal of Marriage and the Family* 46 (1984): 43–55.

49. Bolton, *The Pregnant Adolescent,* 49.

50. Warren B. Miller, "Psychological Vulnerability to Unplanned Pregnancy," *Family Planning Perspectives* 5 (1973): 199–201.

51. A. Johnson and S. Szurek, "The Genesis of Antisocial Acting Out in Children and Adults," *Psychoanalytic Quarterly* 21 (1952): 322–43.

52. C. M. Friedman, R. Greenspan, and F. Mittleman, "The Decision-Making Process and the Outcome of Therapeutic Abortion," *American Journal of Psychiatry* 131 (1974): 1332–37; M. L. Glasser and R. O. Pasnau, "The Unplanned Pregnancy in Adolescence," *The Journal of Family Practice* 2:2 (1975): 91–4.

53. J. M. Low and B. E. Moely, *Difference in Responses to a Behavioral Intervention Program: Older and Younger Pregnant Adoles-*

cents (Paper Presented at the First Biennial Meeting of the Society for Research on Adolescence, Madison, Wis.).

54. Donald R. Atkinson, A. Winzelberg, and A. Holland, "Ethnicity, Locus of Control for Family Planning, and Pregnancy Counselor Credibility," *Journal of Counseling Psychology* 32 (1985): 417–21.

55. M. W. Hanson, "Abortion in Teenagers," *Clinical Obstetrics and Gynecology* 21 (1978): 1175–90.

56. Nathan W. Ackerman, "Sexual Delinquency Among Middle-class Girls," *Family Dynamics and Female Sexual Delinquency* (Palo Alto, Calif.: Science and Behavioral Books, 1969).

57. David A. Baptiste, Jr., "Counseling the Pregnant Adolescent Within a Family Context: Therapeutic Issues and Strategies," *Family Therapy* 13 (1986): 161–176 (quotes found 168–9).

58. Bolton, *The Pregnant Adolescent.*

59. Ibid.

60. Fisher and Ury, *Getting to Yes.*

61. Francis Schaeffer and C. Everett Koop, *What Ever Happened to the Human Race?* (Old Tappan, N.J.: Fleming H. Revell, 1979); C. Marshner, "Once Conceived, A Child Has the Right to Be Born," in Harold and Margaret Feldman, eds., *Current Controversies in Marriage and Family* (Beverly Hills: Sage, 1985), 203–11.

62. Eva Leveton, *Adolescent Crisis: Family Counseling Approaches* (New York: Springer, 1984).

63. Worthington, *Counseling Married Christian Couples* (Downers Grove, Ill.: InterVarsity Press, 1987) in press.

64. Jacquelin S. Kasun, "Teenage Pregnancy: Media Effects Versus Facts," in F. Glahe and J. Peden, eds., *American Family and the State* (San Francisco: Pacific Institute for Policy Research, 1984).

65. A danger that Christians need to be aware of is that definitions of *moral* sex education can differ widely and encompass what many Christians might consider even anti-Christian morals. As an example of this see Sol Gordon, "The Case for a Moral Sex Education in the Schools," *The Journal of School and Health* 51 (1981): 214–8; in which Gordon advocates full knowledge of sexual practices and birth control procedures modeled on sex education programs of Sweden, examination of ethical attitudes to abortion, premarital sex with a person one intends to marry, and acceptance of a variety of means of sexual expression.

66. Roosa, *et al.,* "A Comparison of Teenage and Older Mothers."

67. Erma Bombeck, *If Life Is a Bowl of Cherries, What Am I Doing in the Pits?* (New York: McGraw-Hill, 1971).

Notes

68. Cosby, *Fatherhood*.

69. M. H. Klaus and J. H. Kennell, *Maternal-Infant Bonding: The Impact of Early Separation or Loss on Family Development* (St. Louis: Mosby, 1976).

70. Andrew J. Cherlin, *Marriage, Divorce, Remarriage* (Cambridge, Mass.: Harvard University Press, 1981).

71. Bolton, *The Pregnant Adolescent*.

72. See Roosa *et al.* for a review.

Chapter 5 Cohabiting . . . and Pregnant

1. Graham B. Spanier, "Married and Unmarried Cohabitation in the United States: 1980," *Journal of Marriage and the Family* 45 (1983): 277–88.

2. E. D. Macklin, "Review of Research on Non-Marital Cohabitation in The United States," in B. J. Murstein, eds., *Exploring Intimate Lifestyles* (New York: Springer, 1978).

3. Roy E. L. Watson, "Premarital Cohabitation vs. Traditional Courtship: Their Effects on Subsequent Marital Adjustment," *Family Relations* 32 (1983): 139–47.

4. Spanier, "Married and Unmarried Cohabitation in the United States."

5. For example R. H. Rubin, "It Is Important That Both Men and Women Have Premarital Sex, Especially with the Person They Are Considering for Marriage," in Feldman, *Current Controversies in Marriage and Family*, 45–55; however, not all agree, such as Carlfred B. Broderick, "Both Males and Females Should Be Virgins at the Time of Marriage," in Feldman, *Current Controversies in Marriage and Family*, 37–44.

6. Brigitte Berger and Peter L. Berger, *The War Over the Family: Capturing the Middle Ground* (Garden City, N.Y.: Anchor Press/Doubleday, 1984).

7. I. Hutchinson, *The American Family* (working paper prepared under the sponsorship of the National Council on Family Relations in Preparation for the 1980 White House Conference on Families).

8. Kohlberg, "Revisions in the Theory and Practice of Moral Development."

9. Worthington, Donald B. Danser, Matthew McTaggart, and Sara Beck, *Adolescents' and Their Families' Values Concerning Cohabitation and Religion* (unpublished raw data, 1986).

263

10. Worthington, and Donald B. Danser, "Effects of Late Adolescent's Definition of Cohabitation, Religious Intensity, and Perceived Parent Values on Their Willingness to Engage in Heterosexual Cohabitation," *International Review of Natural Family Planning* (in press).

11. Sources for Table 3: Peter M. Bentler and Michael D. Newcomb, "Longitudinal Study of Marital Success and Failure," *Journal of Consulting and Clinical Psychology* 46 (1978): 1053–70. J. M. Jacques and K. J. Chason, "Cohabitation: Its Impact on Marital Success," *The Family Coordinator* 28 (1979): 35–9. Michael D. Newcomb and Peter M. Bentler, "Assessment of Personality and Demographic Aspects of Cohabitation and Marital Success," *Journal of Personality Assessment* 44 (1980a): 11–24. Michael D. Newcomb and Peter M. Bentler, "Cohabitation Before Marriage: A Comparison of Married Couples Who Did and Did Not Cohabitate," *Alternative Lifestyles* 3 (1980): 65–85. Alfred DeMaris, "A Comparison of Remarriages with First Marriages on Satisfaction in Marriage and Its Relationship to Prior Cohabitation," *Family Relations* 33 (1984): 443–49. Alfred DeMaris and G. R. Leslie, "Cohabitation with the Future Spouse: Its Influence Upon Marital Satisfaction and Communication," *Journal of Marriage and The Family* 46 (1984): 77–84. R.E.L. Watson, "Premarital Cohabitation vs. Traditional Courtship, Their Effects on Subsequent Marital Adjustment," *Family Relations* 32 (1983) 139–47.

12. Michael D. Newcomb, "Heterosexual Cohabitation Relationships," in S. Duck and R. Gilmour, eds., *Personal Relationships 1: Studying Personal Relationships* (London: Academic Press, 1981), 131–64.

13. Cherlin, *Marriage, Divorce, Remarriage.*

14. Watson, "Premarital Cohabitation vs. Traditional Courtship."

15. Worthington *et al.*, *Adolescents and Their Families' Values.*

16. M. Kotkin, "To Marry or Live Together?" *Lifestyles: A Journal of Changing Patterns* 7 (1985): 156–69.

17. Newcomb, "Heterosexual Cohabitation Relationships."

18. John White, *Eros Defiled: The Christian and Sexual Sin* (Downers Grove, Ill.: InterVarsity Press, 1977).

19. Worthington and Buston, "The Marriage Relationship in the Transition to Parenthood."

20. Jay Belsky and Michael Rovine, "Social-network Contact, Family Support, and the Transition to Parenthood," *Journal of Marriage and The Family* 46 (1984): 455–62.

21. Hamilton I. McCubbin and Joan M. Patterson, "Family Transitions: Adaptation to Stress," in Hamilton I. McCubbin and Charles R. Figley, eds., *Stress and the Family: Volume I, Coping with Normative Transitions* (New York: Brunner/Mazel, 1983), 5–25.

22. D. A. Bagarozzi and P. Raven, "Premarital Counseling: Appraisal and Status," *American Journal of Family Therapy* 9(3) (1981): 13–30.

23. Leanne Payne, *The Broken Image: Restoring Personal Wholeness Through Healing Prayer* (Westchester, Ill.: Crossway Books, 1981); L. Rebecca Propst, "A Comparison of the Cognitive Restructuring Psychotherapy Paradigm and Several Spiritual Approaches to Mental Health," *Journal of Psychology and Theology* 8 (1980b): 107–14; Agnes Sanford, *The Healing Light*, rev. ed. (Plainfield, N.J.: Logos, 1972); David A. Seamands, *Healing of Memories* (Wheaton, Ill.: Victor Books, 1985); Ruth Carter Stapleton, *The Gift of Inner Healing* (Waco, Tex.: Word, 1976).

24. Kohlberg, "Revisions in the Theory and Practice of Moral Development."

Chapter 6 Pregnant Newlyweds

1. Boston Women's Health Book Collective, *Ourselves and Our Children: A Book by and for Parents* (New York: Random House, 1978), 34.

2. R. Seiden-Miller, "The Social Construction and Reconstruction of Physiological Events: Acquiring the Pregnancy Identity," *Studies in Symbolic Interaction* 1 (1978): 181–204.

3. Ralph LaRossa, *Becoming a Parent* (Beverly Hills, Calif.: Sage, 1986).

4. Rossi, "Transition to Parenthood."

5. J. M. Hanford, "Pregnancy as a State of Conflict," *Psychological Reports* 22 (1968): 1313–42.

6. M. Leifer, *Psychological Effects of Motherhood: A Study of First Pregnancy* (New York: Praeger, 1980).

7. Cosby, *Fatherhood*, 27.

8. See Shirley M. H. Hanson and Frederick W. Bozett, *Dimensions of Fatherhood* (Beverly Hills, Calif.: Sage 1985) and Bryan E. Robinson and Robert L. Barret, *The Developing Father: Emerging Roles in Contemporary Society* (New York: Guilford, 1986) for a more complete account of the effects of pregnancy on fathers.

9. Anne Campbell and Worthington, "A Comparison of Two Methods of Training Husbands to Assist Their Wives With Labor and Delivery," *Journal of Psychosomatic Research* 25 (1981): 557–63; Anne Campbell and Worthington, "Teaching Expectant Fathers How to Be Better Childbirth Coaches," *MCN, The American Journal of Maternal Child Nursing* 7 (1982): 28–32; Worthington, "Labor Room and Laboratory: Clinical Validation of the Cold Pressor as a Means of Testing Preparation for Childbirth Strategies," *Journal of Psychosomatic Research* 26 (1982): 223–30; Worthington, and Glen A. Martin, "A Laboratory Analysis of Response to Pain After Training in Three Lamaze Techniques," *Journal of Psychosomatic Research* 24 (1980): 109–16; Worthington, Glen A. Martin, Michael Shumate, "Which Prepared Childbirth Coping Strategies Are Effective?," *Journal of Obstetric, Gynecologic, and Neonatal Nursing* 77 (1982): 45–51; Worthington, Glen A. Martin, Michael Shumate, and Johnice Carpenter, "The Effect of Brief Lamaze Training and Social Encouragement on Pain Endurance in a Cold Pressor Task," *Journal of Applied Social Psychology* 13 (1983): 223–33.

10. Worthington and Martin, "A Laboratory Analysis of Response to Pain After Training in Three Lamaze Techniques."

11. Howard J. Markman and F. S. Kadushin, "The Preventative Effects of Lamaze Training for First Time Parents: A Longitudinal Study" (unpublished manuscript, University of Denver, 1983).

12. LaRossa, *Becoming a Parent.*

13. R. Warshaw, "The American Way of Birth," *Ms.* 13 (Sept., 1984): 45–50, 130.

14. For a summary see LaRossa, *Becoming a Parent.*

15. L. Kovit, "Labor Is Hard Work: Notes on the Social Organization of Childbirth," *Sociological Symposium* 8 (Spring, 1972): 11–21.

16. See LaRossa, *Becoming a Parent*, for a review of the history of attitudes toward children.

17. LaRossa, *Becoming a Parent.*

18. Olson, McCubbin *et al., Families.*

19. Worthington and Buston, "The Marriage Relationship in the Transition to Parenthood."

20. Myers-Walls, "Balancing Multiple Role Responsibilities During the Transition to Parenthood."

21. Harriman, "Personal and Marital Changes Accompanying Parenthood."

22. Worthington and Buston, "The Marriage Relationship in the Transition to Parenthood."

23. R. P. Lederman, *Psychosocial Adaptation to Pregnancy: Assessment of Seven Dimensions of Maternal Development* (Englewood Cliffs, N.J.: Prentice-Hall, 1984); P. M. Sherefshefsky and L. Yarrow, *Psychological Aspects of a First Pregnancy* (New York: Raven Press, 1974).

24. L. G. Calhoun, J. W. Selby, and H. E. King, "The Influence of Pregnancy on Sexuality: A Review of Current Evidence," *Journal of Sex Research* 17 (1981): 139–51; Ralph LaRossa, "Sex During Pregnancy: A Symbolic Interactionist Analysis," *Journal of Sex Research* 15 (1979): 119–28.

25. LaRossa, *Becoming a Parent.*

26. V. C. Fox and M. H. Quitt, *Loving, Parenting, and Dying* (New York: Psychohistory Press, 1980).

27. Jay Belsky, M. Perry-Jenkins, and A. C. Crouter, "The Work-Family Interface and Marital Change Across the Transition to Parenthood," *Journal of Family Issues* 6 (1985): 205–20; Doris R. Entwisle and Susan Doering, *The First Birth: A Family Turning Point* (Baltimore, Md.: The Johns Hopkins University Press, 1981).

28. W. A. Goldberg, G. Y. Michaels, and M. E. Lamb, "Husbands' and Wives' Patterns of Adjustment to Pregnancy and First Parenthood," *Journal of Family Issues* 7 (1985): 483–504.

29. W. J. Goode, "A Theory of Role Strain," *American Sociological Review* 25 (1960): 483–96.

30. Worthington and Buston, "The Marriage Relationship in the Transition to Parenthood."

31. For example, recently G. J. Chelune, and E. M. Waring, "Nature and Assessment of Intimacy," in P. McReynolds (ed), *Advances in Psychological Assessment* (San Francisco: Jossey-Bass, 1984); B. Davidson, J. Balswick, and C. Halverson, "Affective Self-Disclosure and Marital Adjustment: A Test of Equity Theory," *Journal of Marriage and the Family* 45 (1983): 93–102; B. E. Tolstedt and J. P. Stokes, "Relation of Verbal, Affective, and Physical Intimacy to Marital Satisfaction," *Journal of Counseling Psychology* 30 (1983): 573–80; E. M. Waring and G. J. Chelune, "Marital Intimacy and Self-Disclosure," *Journal of Clinical Psychology* 39 (1983): 183–90; L. K. White, "Determinants of Spousal Interaction: Marital Structure or Marital Happiness," *Journal of Marriage and the Family* 45 (1983): 511–19.

32. LaRossa, *Becoming a Parent.*

33. J. Scanzoni, "Social Processes and Power in Families," in W. R. Burr *et al.* (eds), *Contemporary Theories About the Family, Volume 1: Research-based Theories* (New York: Free Press, 1979).

34. R. J. Gelles, "Violence and Pregnancy: A Note of the Extent of the Problem and Needed Services," *Family Coordinator* 24 (1975): 81–6; J. Giles-Sims, *Wife-Battering: A Systems Theory Approach* (New York: Guilford, 1983).

35. Argyle and Furnham, "Sources of Satisfaction and Conflict in Long-term Relationships"; Jacobson, Waldron, and Moore, "Toward a Behavioral Profile of Marital Distress."

36. Worthington, "Effects of Marriage Happiness and Duration of Marriage on Conflict, Emotional Climate, Cluster Stress, and Triangulation in Marriage: A Preliminary Test of Two of Guerin's Stages of Marital Disharmony" (unpublished manuscript, Virginia Commonwealth University, 1986).

37. Thomas H. Holmes and R. H. Rahe, "The Social Readjustment Rating Scale," *Journal of Psychosomatic Research* 11 (1967): 213–18.

38. Hamilton I. McCubbin and Joan M. Patterson, "Family Adaptation to Crisis," in Hamilton McCubbin, A. Cauble, and Joan M. Patterson, eds., *Family Stress, Coping and Social Support* (Springfield, Ill.: Charles C. Thomas, 1982).

39. LaRossa, *Becoming a Parent*.

40. Worthington, Beverley G. Buston, and T. Michael Hammonds, "A Component Analysis of Marriage Enrichment: Information and Social Support," (unpublished manuscript, Virginia Commonwealth University, 1986).

41. Worthington, *Counseling Married Christian Couples*.

42. Myers-Walls, "Balancing Multiple Role Responsibilities During the Transition to Parenthood."

43. Brent C. Miller and D. Sollie, "Normal Stresses During the Transition to Parenthood," *Family Relations* 29 (1980): 459–65.

Chapter 7 Back-to-Back Children

1. Elizabeth Noble, *Having Twins: A Parent's Guide to Pregnancy, Birth, and Early Childhood* (Boston: Houghton-Mifflin, 1980).

2. Noble, *Having Twins*.

3. M. Gaddis, and V. Gaddis, *The Curious World of Twins* (New York: Warner, 1973); A. Smith, *The Body* (New York: Walker and Company, 1968); R. T. Theroux, and J. F. Tingley, *The Care of Twin Children* (Chicago: Center for Study of Multiple Gestation, 1978).

4. See Noble, *Having Twins,* for a list of recommended readings.

5. E. A. Schaughency, and B. B. Lahey, "Mothers' and Fathers' Perceptions of Child Deviance: Roles of Child Behavior, Parental Depression, and Marital Satisfaction," *Journal of Consulting and Clinical Psychology* 53 (1985): 718–23.

6. Ann Kiemel Anderson, and J. Kiemel Ream, *Struggling for Wholeness* (Nashville: Oliver-Nelson Books, 1986).

Chapter 8 Thy Quiver Overfloweth

1. LaRossa, *Becoming a Parent.*

2. R. J. Gelles, and C. P. Cornell, *Intimate Violence in Families* (Beverly Hills, Calif.: Sage, 1985).

3. J. Kirkland, "Infant Crying—Problem That Won't Go Away!" *Parents' Centre Bulletin* 96 (1983): 15–7; J. Kirkland, F. Deane, and M. Brennan, "About CrySOS, A Clinic for People with Crying Babies," *Family Relations* 32 (1983): 537–43.

4. Virginia Apgar, and Joan Beck, *Is My Baby All Right?* (New York: Trident Press, 1973).

5. Ibid.

6. Ibid.

7. Ibid.

8. Ibid.

9. Ibid.

10. Klaus and Kennell, *Maternal-Infant Bonding: The Impact of Early Separation or Loss on Family Development;* A. J. Solnit, and M. Stark, "Mourning the Birth of a Defective Child," *Psychoanalytic Study of Children* 16 (1961): 523–37.

11. L. Wikler, "Chronic Stresses of Families of Mentally Retarded Children," *Family Relations* 30 (1981): 281–8.

12. Joan M. Patterson and Hamilton I. McCubbin, "Chronic Illness: Family Stress and Coping," in Charles R. Figley and Hamilton I. McCubbin, *Stress and the Family: Volume II, Coping with Catastrophe* (New York: Brunner/Mazel, 1983), 21–36.

13. See Patterson and McCubbin, "Chronic Illness: Family Stress and Coping" for a summary of the different tasks of the family throughout the life cycle of the handicapped or chronically ill child.

14. C. S. Lewis, "God in the Dock," in W. Hooper, ed., *God in the Dock: Essays on Theology and Ethics* (Grand Rapids, Mich.: Eerdmans, 1970), 240–4.

15. M. Shere, "The Social-Emotional Development of the Twin Who Has Cerebral Palsy," *Cerebral Palsy Review* 17 (1957): 16–8.

16. V. Cardwell, *Cerebral Palsy: Advances in Understanding and Care* (New York: Association for the Aid of Crippled Children, 1956).

17. R. Darling, *Families Against Society: A Study of Reaction to Children with Birth Defects* (Beverly Hills, Calif.: Sage, 1979).

18. P. Chodoff, S. Friedman, and D. Hamburg, "Stress Defenses and Six Coping Behaviors: Observations in Parents of Children with Malignant Disease," *American Journal of Psychiatry* 120(8) (1964): 734–49.

19. Hamilton I. McCubbin, M. McCubbin, R. Nevin, and E. Cauble, *CHIP—Coping Health Inventory for Parents* (St. Paul: Family Social Science, 1979).

20. Hamilton I. McCubbin, M. McCubbin, Joan M. Patterson, E. Cauble, L. Wilson, and W. Warwick, "CHIP—Coping Health Inventory for Parents: An Assessment of Parental Coping Patterns in the Case of the Chronically Ill Child," *Journal of Marriage and the Family* (1984).

Chapter 9 Unexpected Midlife Pregnancies

1. J. DeFrain, L. Martens, J. Stork, and W. Stork, *Stillborn: The Invisible Death* (Lexington, Mass.: Lexington Books, 1986).

2. R. Brent, and M. Harris, eds., *Prevention of Embryonic, Fetal, and Perinatal Disease* DHEW. Publication No. (NIH) 76–853 (Bethesda, Md.: National Institutes of Health, 1976).

3. G. L. Rubin, H. B. Peterson, S. F. Dorfman, *et al.*, "Ectopic Pregnancy in the United States: 1970 through 1978," *Journal of the American Medical Association* 249 (1983): 1725–29.

4. J. A. Merrill, "Endometriosis," in D. Danforth (ed), *Obstetrics and Gynecology* 4th ed. (Philadelphia: Harper and Row, 1982), 1004–14.

5. J. A. Pritchard, and P. C. MacDonald, *Williams Obstetrics* 16th ed. (New York: Appleton-Century-Crofts, 1976).

6. Ibid.

7. J. B. Hardy, and E. D. Mellits, "Relationship of Low Birth Weight to Maternal Characteristics of Age, Parity, Education, and Body Size," in D. M. Reed and F. J. Stanley, eds., *The Epidemiology of Prematurity* (proceedings of a working conference at NICH D-NIH, Bethesda, Md., November 1976; Baltimore and Munich: Urban and Schwaizenburg, 1977).

8. S. P. Rubin, *It's Not Too Late for a Baby: For Men and Women Over 35* (Englewood Cliffs, N.J.: Prentice-Hall, 1980).

9. P. Placek, S. Taffel, and M. Moien, "Caesarean Section Delivery Rates: United States, 1981," *American Journal of Public Health* 73 (1983): 861–2.

10. J. B. Cohen, *Parenthood After 30? A Guide to Personal Choice* (Lexington, Mass.: Lexington Books, 1985).

11. Z. Stein, and J. Kline, "Smoking, Alcohol, and Reproduction," *American Journal of Public Health* 73 (1983): 1154–56; D. U. Himmelberger, B. W. Brown, Jr., and E. N. Cohen, "Cigarette Smoking During Pregnancy and the Occurrence of Spontaneous Abortion and Congenital Abnormality," *American Journal of Epidemiology* 108 (1978): 470–9; J. Kline, and Z. Stein, M. Susser, *et al.*, "Smoking: A Risk Factor for Spontaneous Abortion," *New England Journal of Medicine* 297 (1977): 793–6.

12. E. B. Hook and E. M. Chambers, "Estimated Rates of Down's Syndrome in Live Births by One Year Maternalize Intervals for Mothers Aged 20–29 in a New York State Study," in D. Bergsma and B. R. Lowry (eds), *Numerical Taxonomy and Polygenic Disorders* (New York: National Foundation—March of Dimes, 1977), 123–41.

13. National Institute of Child Health and Human Development, National Institutes of Health, *Antenatal Diagnosis: Report of a Consensus Development Conference* (Washington, D.C.: U.S. Department of Health, Education and Welfare, 1979).

14. Cohen, *Parenthood After 30?*

15. Ibid.

16. DeFrain *et al.*, *Stillborn.*

17. LaRossa, *Becoming a Parent.*

18. DeFrain *et al.*, *Stillborn.*

19. Ibid., 121.

20. C. A. Walter, *The Timing of Motherhood* (Lexington, Mass.: Lexington Books, 1985).

21. DeFrain *et al.*, *Stillborn.*

Chapter 10 Counseling the Infertile Couple

1. Anne Martin Matthews, and Ralph Matthews, "Infertility and Involuntary Childlessness: Beyond the Mechanics of Infertility," *Family Relations*, in press; Anne Martin Matthews, and Ralph Matthews, "Perspectives on Infertility and Involuntary Childlessness: Beyond the Mechanics of Infertility," *Family Relations*, in press;

Ralph Matthews, and Anne Martin Matthews, "Infertility and Involuntary Childlessness: The Transition to Nonparenthood," *Journal of Marriage and the Family* 48 (1986): 641–9.

2. A. M. Matthews and R. Matthews, "Infertility and Involuntary Childlessness," 642.

3. J. A. Stigger, *Coping with Infertility: A Guide for Couples, Families, and Counselors* (Minneapolis: Augsburg, 1983).

4. Ibid.

5. Barbara Eck-Menning, *Infertility: A Guide for the Childless Couple* (Englewood Cliffs, N.J.: Prentice-Hall, 1977); Stigger, *Coping With Infertility*; M. Stout, *Without Child: A Compassionate Look at Infertility* (Grand Rapids, Mich.: Zondervan, 1985); R. Matthews and A. M. Matthews, "Infertility and Involuntary Childlessness"; Diana Burguryn, *Marriage Without Children* (New York: Harper and Row, 1981); William H. James, "Has Fecundity Been Declining in Recent Years in Developed Countries?" *Journal of Biosocial Science* 13 (1981): 419–24.

6. Stigger, *Coping with Infertility.*

7. Ibid.

8. A. M. Matthews, and R. Matthews, "Infertility and Involuntary Childlessness."

9. Ibid.

10. Stigger, *Coping with Infertility*; Stout, *Without Child.*

11. Sheldon Stryker, "Identity Salience and Role Performance: The Relevance of Symbolic Interaction for Family Research," *Journal of Marriage and the Family* 30 (1968): 558–64; Sheldon Stryker, *Symbolic Interactionism* (Menlo Park, Calif.: Benjamin-Cummings, 1980).

12. Charlene E. Miall, "Self-labeling and the Stigma of Involuntary Childlessness," *Social Problems,* in press.

13. A. M. Matthews and R. Matthews, "Infertility and Involuntary Childlessness."

14. Marvin B. Scott and Stanford M. Lyman, "Accounts," *American Sociological Review* 33 (1968): 46–62.

15. Eck-Menning, *Infertility*; Adrienne D. Kraft, J. Palombo, D. Mitchell, C. Dean, S. Meyers, and A. W. Schmidt, "The Psychological Dimensions of Infertility," *American Journal of Orthopsychiatry* 50 (1962): 618–28; Karen S. Renne, "Childlessness, Health, and Marital Satisfaction," *Social Biology* 23 (1976): 183–97.

16. Trudy Bradley, *An Exploration of Caseworker's Perceptions of Adoptive Applicants* (New York: Child Welfare League of America, 1967); Child Welfare League of America, *Standards for Adop-*

tion Service, rev. ed. (New York: Author, 1978); Joan McNamara, *The Adoption Advisor* (New York: Hawthorn, 1975).

17. Stigger, *Coping with Infertility.*
18. Stout, *Without Child.*
19. Stigger, *Coping with Infertility.*
20. Stout, *Without Child.*
21. Stigger, *Coping with Infertility.*

Chapter 11 Who's in Control Here?

1. The other three are Worthington, *When Someone Asks for Help* (Downers Grove, Ill.: InterVarsity Press, 1984; Worthington, *How to Help the Hurting: When Friends Face Problems with Self-Esteem, Self Control, Fear, Depression, Loneliness* (Downers Grove, Ill.: InterVarsity Press, 1985); Worthington, *Counseling Married Christian Couples* (Downers Grove, Ill.: InterVarsity Press, in press).

2. H. S. Kushner, *When Bad Things Happen to Good People* (New York: Avon, 1981).

3. C. S. Lewis, *The Problem of Pain* (New York: Macmillan, 1962), 93.

INDEX

Everett L. Worthington, Jr., Ph.D.

Everett Worthington is associate professor of psychology at the Virginia Commonwealth University. He has authored numerous scholarly research articles and has written three books, *When Someone Asks for Help, How to Help the Hurting,* and *Marriage Counseling with Christian Couples.* Having received the B.S. at the University of Tennessee and the M.S. at Massachusetts Institute of Technology, both in nuclear engineering, he held a commission in the U.S. Navy and served as an instructor in the Naval Nuclear Power School. Dr. Worthington subsequently earned the M.A. and Ph.D. degrees in counseling psychology at the University of Missouri. He and his wife Kirby live in Richmond, Virginia, and are the parents of four children, Christen, Jonathan, Becca, and Katy Anna.